VOYA
through
THE MIST

an emotional journey of life, love and learning

by
Jane Seaman

MWI Publishing

Published in Great Britain 2011
by

MASTERWORKS INTERNATIONAL
27 Old Gloucester Street
London
WC1N 3XX
UK

Email: admin@mwipublishing.com
Web: http://www.mwipublishing.com

ISBN: 978-0-9565803-1-3

Book cover by Mywizarddesign.com
Cover image: Shaman's bowl from Antaratma/Dreamstime.com

All rights reserved. No part of this book or other material may be reproduced in any form without written permission of the publishers.

Copyright © 2011, Jane Seaman

Contents

SHADES OF BLUE
5

OCEAN BLUE
23

MUDDY WATERS
37

AWAKENING SPRINGS
55

RIPPLING WAVES
69

BREAKING WATER
83

THE BIG SURF
93

TSUNAMI HITS
109

BABBLING BROOKS
127

WHIRLPOOLS
137

INFINITE DEEP WATERS OF LIFE
149

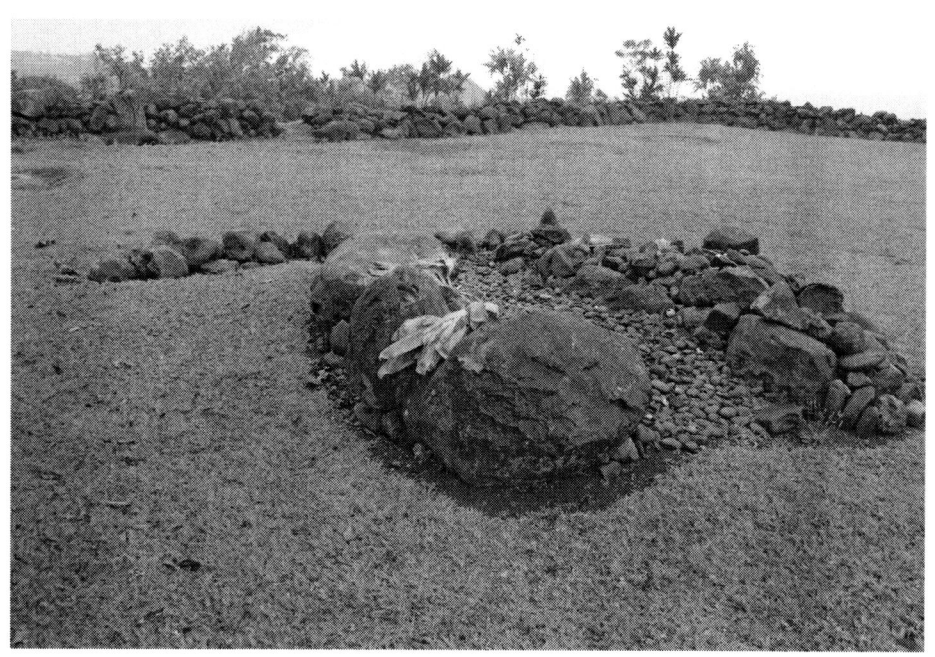

Kukuipuka Heaiu – a divine place of healing and refuge located on a hilltop overlooking the Wailuku region on Maui, Hawaii.

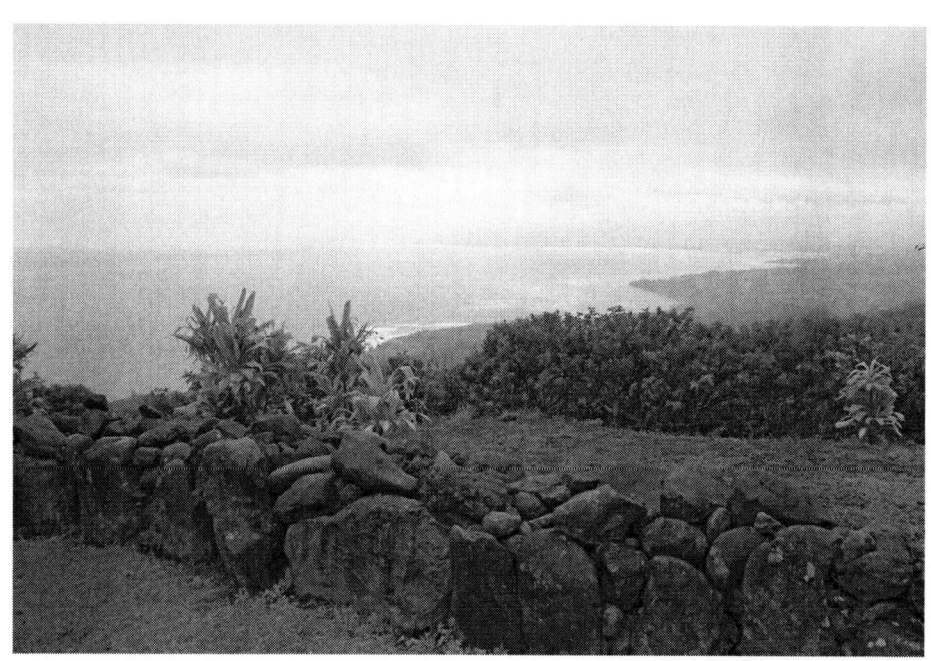

SHADES OF BLUE

"Like a delicate flower, slowly opening as the shades of light begin to show"
Jane Seaman

Confusion reigns

It was a cold December winter's day, I was wrapped up to the nines as my sister and I climbed out of the car. With a sense of dread and fear in the pit of my stomach we entered an old musty smelling village hall. A blast of warm air hit us as we clambered into the room. It was the last ballet class of the term. I was five years old and this was my first experience of performing in front of so many people.

I was desperate. My insides squirmed and I was on the edge of tears as one by one each of us waited our turn to perform on our own. This was a test to see how much we had learned. All I wanted to do was hide away. When it came to my turn, I'd forgotten everything. Holding my breath I froze like a startled animal, wide eyed and unable to move. I can't actually remember if I danced or not.

As we finally left the hall, which for me was for the last time as I wasn't enrolled in any more lessons, I felt like a failure, yet I was hugely relieved that I didn't have to do this anymore. My shyness was intense. Even now thinking about it, I remember just wanting to disappear. People scared me then. I would hide behind my parent's legs if anyone spoke to me. I wouldn't say 'boo' to a goose and go bright red like a beacon. At this very early age, life through my eyes was huge, confusing and frightening.

I remember my early years through a sense of bewilderment. What on earth I am doing here, I would think to myself. I couldn't find the words to articulate how I felt, so when I sensed fearful situations I would cry or hide away. Shyness was to be a blessing as well as a curse in future years.

We lived in a 'well to do' area in the south of the United Kingdom. Our location seemed perfect in many ways. It felt like we were living in the country, surrounded by trees and a huge public green, yet near enough to a mainline railway station and with main roads to the nearest towns. We were about a one hour drive from the metropolis that is London. Our bungalow was built pre the 1930's and it enjoyed a good sized garden with enough ground space to expand the family home in the future. Backed onto our garden were fields and a wood of the tallest Poplar trees I have ever seen. I loved to see them swaying, dancing and whispering in the breeze.

Mum and Dad were decent middle class hard working people. Mum, the youngest from a large family of eleven other brothers and sisters, grew up in a huge family home in the Surrey suburbs. Her father was a manager of a factory, whom she feared, but she has always been full of praise for her mother. Mum was a beautiful lady, five foot three with a lovely smile, petite slim figure and dark brown eyes. I could see from the photographs that we have, that she had been active and full of life. Mum used to love to dance and play tennis, but she was also shy. She had gone on to do well at secretarial school and then enjoyed working for various top class city based firms, before meeting and marrying my Dad. I never knew my Mum as this vivacious lady. She suffered from manic depression and I was to grow up knowing a very different side to her.

Dad stood tall, over six foot, he was slim and agile with green-blue eyes and he was the youngest brother to twin sisters. He was the oracle in our family, full of knowledge and seemed to know everything, domineering, strict, and sociable. Dad didn't take any nonsense, a black and white kind of guy. Growing up as a young boy during the war time, he and his friends would fend for themselves, playing in and around the gravel pits near Heathrow. They would find unexploded incendiary devices and throw them against walls to try and make them detonate , then proceed to squirt pee to make them fizzle, running away in fits of laughter, innocent 'fun' but very dangerous! For the young boys at that time, the war was more exciting than fearful. His father, my Grandfather was in the Navy and ever absent. He would come home on leave, telling exotic and exciting stories about his adventures. Dad relished the short times he spent with his father when he was home on leave. His mother, my Nan, was a tall strict domineering character, a member of the local amateur dramatics club and very hard working. Dad became the 'man of the house' as he grew into a teenager, leaving school at fourteen to take up an apprenticeship in electronics, eventually joining the Royal Electrical Mechanical Engineers and serving in Egypt for his National Service. This is where he developed a passion for mending and building cars and motorbikes. When he completed his National Service, he met and married my mother. At the same time Dad started up his own business as a garage proprietor, took on a mortgage to buy the bungalow and Mum became unexpectedly pregnant with my brother. Dad loved his work, it suited him to be in his element doing something that he was passionate about. Dad could have been anything, extremely intelligent and bright, yet he chose to work with his hands and create magic in fixing and putting things back together. However, life was a struggle in the beginning as they strove to build a life and family home with very little income.

After my brother was born in the late 1950's, just under two years later, my sister, a planned addition to the family arrived and a further two years later, as a surprise, I popped into this world. My mother was distraught. She had become fearful that she may end up like her own mother, having so many children. Mum wasn't naturally a maternal person. After my sister was born, she suffered serious post natal depression, although in those days not much was known about the baby blues. She was still depressed when I was conceived. The last thing she wanted was another baby. But, I arrived into this world one Sunday afternoon in October, extremely quickly and jaundiced. Mum's depression deepened and after many visits to the doctors she was eventually diagnosed with manic depression (bi-polar disorder) and was given many prescription drugs to help even out her mood swings.

We lived in a lovely area, surrounded by beauty. Mum stayed at home to bring us up and Dad did his best to bring in a solid income, to support the growing family. When they bought the house it needed renovation and they worked tirelessly on getting the house into a liveable condition, initially on a very tight budget. Luckily, through his determination, Dads' business thrived.

On one level our life sounded ideal, however for me, my early years seemed such a struggle. I felt very little connection to my Mum, although I wanted to connect, there wasn't anything coming back and nothing seemed to make sense. I didn't feel safe. As I grew into school age, I was told, the school years would be the best years of my life. Yet it didn't feel like that to me. School was a nightmare. I thought life must be better than this and why did I feel so different? I found school boring and restrictive.

My sister was the brainy one apparently. I didn't appear to be an intellectual kid like her, but I was known to do my best and had a good attitude and was practically adept. So much emphasis was placed on learning stuff that simply wasn't very logical to me at the time, just words and figures. I felt trapped, lost concentration and got very bored. I used to think to myself, "I must be useless." Everyone else seemed to love school so why didn't I feel the same?

I didn't do badly as I was in a reasonably high graded class, but inside I didn't feel like I was doing okay at all. It was a duty and for the most part not enjoyable. Some classes were an absolute chore, trying to sit still and concentrate when I had no interest in a particular subject, like maths. I never really got excited at all about the subject and found it hard work. I would feel dumb sometimes and simply couldn't get past the basics in understanding logarithms and the like. I dreaded the class. I didn't realise until many years later, that it is okay to be different. Some children, like me need stimulating at an early age in a different way. It didn't mean that we were any less of value or worthy of great things, we just didn't fit into that particular box of learning.

I really enjoyed and had the ability to take myself to the extreme physically. "Jane's got ants in her pants," I was chided. I lived for sports recreation lessons. I loved to move. I found a real sense of freedom, fun and expression, through joyfully running around outside in the fresh air, being in tune with everything. In amongst the tedium of daily lessons, there were other glimmers of enjoyment at school. I loved geography but that was because we had a cool teacher. Art was also a blessing, as images came into my mind I could blend colour and make pictures look pretty. These three lessons were my saving grace, I gained a sense of perspective and self worth, as they were classes I found easy.

At home, emotional confusion reigned in my family. My Mum was addicted to pills and couldn't survive without her fix. In those days there didn't seem any other way to help her. The doctors knew best in my parent's eyes as they had no other point of reference for help. Coupled with that was a real stigma about any sort of mental disease, people didn't know how to respond, understand or behave towards it.

I didn't understand Mum at all, deeply worried and concerned on one level and anxious about what mood she would be in on another. I was always trying to please, but nothing much would come back at all and I would worry what I had done wrong. All I wanted was a cuddle and to feel safe. I didn't realise until years later that she felt nothing and wasn't able to give back much at all. I sensed we were a nuisance, as Mother would brush us aside and tell us to be quiet or to, "wait until your father comes home!" It must have been awful for her. When she emerged on an upside, positive and happy, it was almost too much the other way. It was so lovely to see. But we would all be waiting for the crash and be anxious about when it would come. We never knew what mood she would be in. So I always sensed tension in the air.

However, in Dad's eyes Mother came first in all things. He doted on her – bought her anything she wished. As depression was becoming better understood in the medical field, Dad took Mum to see some of the best doctors, psychiatrists and hypnotists around. The prescription drugs continued and were a problem. They had to be closely monitored as Mum became dependant on them, and there was no sense of wanting to get her off the drugs.

It was like she wasn't there for us, not able to truly interact or engage. How could she? Her feelings were being suppressed and I would often see her drowsy and lethargic and generally unhappy, locked away in her misery.

In an effort to make her cheerful, my Dad would shower her with gifts. The response was often short lived, but in some ways well worth it to see Mum smile for a while. I never saw much real love or affection between them, the odd hug, but generally that area was controlled by Mum's moods. It took me years to understand that she never really wanted to get well and whilst she was taking drugs that literally numbed the senses, how could she ever break out? She received so much attention by being ill, why change? Ultimately, it doesn't matter how much help you get, it is down to the individual to want to get better and Mum simply didn't.

Depression is such a debilitating condition and a real challenge for anyone to understand if you haven't been through it yourself. Mum's fear was of losing her mind. She would feel so anxious and out of control, a real gut wrenching fear, completely incapacitating her. The pills kept this feeling at bay, but it left her like a zombie. Mum feared even the thought of coming off them and to confirm this fear a doctor once told her she would never do so. What a thing to say to someone! That was all she needed to hear, as far as she was concerned she would never come off the drugs, the doctor had said so. She thought it would kill her, if she did. In her eyes there was no hope.

As a child, I struggled to understand. To be told, "Mummy's not well, be quiet, leave her alone" and to be constantly wondering why she was always going to the doctors was difficult. Worry and anxiousness became a natural state for me. All I wanted was to be loved, hugged and cherished by my Mum. I never knew a mother's love and would often look at other parents and children interacting together and think what had I done wrong?

Control

The eldest of the three of us, was my brother Robert. He found a way to stay out of it all. He somehow detached from the emotion and occasionally became my protector during the fights I had with my sister. Robert was liked by everyone. He was relatively shy also, tall with jet black hair. Not a stranger to being bullied, he was teased at school for wearing glasses and called 'four eyes' and other similarly unpleasant words by the other school kids. It never seemed to really bother him. He would just brush it off and let it go. Robert was discovered to be dyslexic. They only realised this later on in his schooling years, so he had struggled through for many years in normal lessons, not being recognised for who he really was. Robert was a happy boy, loved to laugh and seemed to keep out of any trouble brewing in the family. Even though he was four years older than me, I felt protective of Robert and I got on well with him and often felt a subtle level of understanding between us that was unspoken, but always there.

Gillian my sister was the bully, two years older than me, very angry and a complete polarity to me in almost every way. She never bullied my brother. I was the easy target, younger, weaker and didn't know how to defend myself against her anger and aggression. I was a weakling in her eyes. Gillian was an inch taller than me at five foot five, long chestnut brown hair and brown eyes, slim with plenty of attitude. Dogmatic and domineering, you wouldn't want to cross her. She was rebellious and would do everything opposite to what was asked. She clashed with my Dad. What a challenge for my parents, particularly my mother, who was not able to deal with any emotional turmoil, not even her own.

My relationship with Gillian compounded my insecurities and battered me in all directions in the early years. She would generally start the fights, out of the blue, would pull my hair for no reason, pinch me, attack me verbally and viciously and wait for me in the school playground to continue the deluge of abuse. No wonder I hated school! When she had nothing to do, I would be the target. I think most of my early school years were spent in tears, trying to pull myself together in the classroom following a ten minute session of being caught in the corner of the playground with my sister and her friends all in on the act. I didn't have the inner resources to cope.

I felt terrible most of the time. Abuse is an awful thing. It knocks the stuffing out of you; makes you feel the lowest of the low; depletes you so much there is no strength or the state of mind to fight back. The spirit is literally battered out of the way. The words would hurt more than the physical abuse. It made me feel worthless. I had no understanding why anyone could do this to another person and I often felt completely alone – fighting for survival. I didn't know how to articulate or express my feelings at the time. How could I tell anyone? I felt weak and thought I was insignificant. I can hear the answers. "Stand up for yourself." "Don't be silly, she's only playing and doesn't mean it." Only the 'playing' got worse. Eventually and thankfully Mum and Dad recognised this as a serious problem, for both my sister and me.

Gillian and I shared a bedroom and sometimes that was hell as there was nowhere for me to get away. There were snippets of light and laughter. We occasionally would play like two 'normal' sisters and have great fun. I remember one Sunday morning my sister and I rolled ourselves up in our blankets, like sausage rolls and hid at the end of the bed. It was exciting at the time as it looked like we were up and out of bed. We thought we were being clever and couldn't be seen rolled up at the end of the bed. We giggled. I've always been able to giggle at the slightest opportunity. It felt like we were partners in crime for once. Of course, we were found out and told it wasn't very clever, not to be so stupid and to get up, get dressed and make the bed. Silly really, but that's what kids do isn't it, act silly?

I was a skinny kid, my hair which was blond and curly had started to fall out. My hair became dead straight and turned a light brown later on. I really disliked the food at school and hardly ate anything. I particularly didn't like eating meat. My parents were concerned and, in their infinite wisdom and without really understanding my inner turmoil, made me sit at the table and not leave until I had eaten the meat. My parents didn't know any different and thought this was for the best – they worried that I wasn't getting any protein, so I must eat meat.

I didn't like the taste of meat and making me eat it made the situation worse. My saving grace was our dog Minnie, a lovely natured black and white mongrel. I remember, she would patiently wait by my chair. She, of course, knew what was to come! I would chew and chew a mouthful of meat and then carefully, I would spit the mashed up meat into my hand and give it to her under the table. Phew! Then I would feel guilty as I knew it wasn't allowed to feed the dog at the table. Anxiety would bubble up as I knew I had done wrong and feared being found out!

So eating food became a real problem for me as a young child. Most embarrassingly, my parents wrote to the school to ask for special dispensation for me to bring in sandwiches as I didn't eat school lunches. It was the smell and sight of the dinners which put me off. In some ways, this was even worse, now I was being separated from the rest. To cap it all, I would only eat banana sandwiches! This provided more ammunition for the big girls, meaning my sister and her entourage, to bully me. Amazingly in my own age group I had no problem with bullies. Although incredibly naïve, I was part of the 'in crowd' in my year at school. This felt good as I belonged to something that was 'cool.'

Finally, after many horrible and distressing episodes with my sister, Dad decided to separate us. He converted the loft into a bedroom. I cannot tell you what a huge relief this was and the sanctuary that this became. At last I was able to retreat to a space that was my own. My sister was not allowed up and I was not allowed in her room. It was heaven and an adventure. I had my own special stairway, a loft ladder with a hatch. Awesome! I felt special!

Surface tension

Life went on, Mum and Dad strived to provide for us and ensure we had a socially acceptable family unit. His business went from strength to strength. In his no nonsense way, Dad commanded respect. He was in control, honest, talented, intelligent and opinionated. Dad always said if he couldn't make a living working five days a week, between eight thirty and five thirty then he would give up and work for someone else. His priority was supporting the family. I came to remember those wise words years later. This really did give us a sense of security on the outside, yet no one knew of the emotional insecurity and complete contrast that went on at home.

I never heard my parents argue, although there were lots of silences. I am sure that's where I learned how to tune into my sixth sense, knowing when things weren't quite right. Yet it did not stop me worrying about what it was that didn't feel right. Emotions and feelings were not articulated in front of us. Mother seemed to feel awful most of the time so that we became very sensitive to her moods and adapted accordingly. I would often think mother hated me. She seemed to blame us for her feeling bad.

Routine was the order of the day and worked around Dad's work times. He would spend his first half an hour from work at home 'switching off.' We all knew not to disturb him too much during this time as he could have a sharp tongue. It must have been particularly difficult for Mum, as she very often couldn't cope with our childlike outbursts and threatened us many times with, "Be quiet, just wait till your father gets home." Of course, I would quake in my shoes waiting for Dad to come home, wondering if I had done something wrong, more often than not though, it was my sister who was in trouble!

There were elements of structure in our household and we would get together as a family at mealtimes and to enjoy family entertainment. We were encouraged to play a musical instrument. My sister and I started off with the recorder. Mum was a great piano player and both my parents became interested in leaning to play the organ. Dad learned from scratch and Mum transferred her skills easily and naturally. My brother played the trumpet in a band and at times we would all get together and create some sort of noise that resembled a piece of music. Later, both my sister and I learned to play the organ too.

In amongst my Mother' depressive times, she created some great tasting food, when she wanted to. She loved to make fairy cakes and would ensure that there was a meal on the table at the right time for when Dad came home. Our meals, although tasty, would be more often than not predictable and according to the day of the week. Mondays, was left over's from Sunday lunch with bubble and squeak; Tuesdays, cauliflower cheese; Wednesdays stew and dumplings; Thursdays a surprise, maybe cottage pie or something, and Fridays fish and chips, Saturdays maybe spaghetti or chops and smashed potato with vegetables.

In her own agony of despair, Mother started to drink sherry. Her feelings already numbed by prescription drugs, this seemed yet another escape. She already smoked up to forty cigarettes a day. I hated the cigarette smoke and when both Mum and Dad lit up, I would tense up. It felt icky, choked me and made everything smell horrible. The living room would be thick with smoke. I couldn't breathe.

I avoided bringing any friends round to the house as I couldn't be sure if Mum would be okay or not. I had one special friend Katie. She understood and was always there for me. Her family seemed normal and I enjoyed going round to her house to play.

I am sorry to say that I was afraid of my Mum, as I never knew what mood she would be in. How would people understand, much better they didn't know at all. What if she had been drinking, what if she was depressed? If she was in one of her moods it would make me feel awful too and I would be on tenterhooks. Katie seemed not to worry about all of that, she was my best friend. I was so nervous and shy socially, yet I had so much energy inside. Thank goodness I could channel that energy into sports. Apart from my sister and her groupies, I was generally liked at school and at the clubs that I became part of later. No one really knew the lack of self worth I felt inside. I tried not to offend anyone and would endeavour to do my best at everything.

The fear of travelling

Never a great car traveller, I always ended up being car sick. The combination of cigarette smoke in a closed environment with the motion of the car was unbearable. At the weekends we would travel down to the seaside, as both my parents liked to fish. I loved being by the ocean. For me, it was bliss, the fresh air and ever changing scenery. Dreading the car ride, but looking forward to the treat at the end, I would sit by the window 'just in case' I was sick.

Inevitably I would hold on until about thirty minutes travelling time was left. "Stop," I would wail, "I am going to be sick!" The car would stop and I'd fall out the door and retch my guts up. It was horrible.

Then the backlash of teasing from my sister, "Urgh, you smell, get away, what a cretin." Once at the seaside, I would fall out of the car again, breathe and begin to feel my feet on the ground – absolute bliss. My parents were from a generation where smoking was an acceptable social activity and it must have been difficult for them to understand why I despised it so much. Years later they both stopped through serious illness.

In spite of all of my own personal sensitivities as a child, my parents were good people, just caught up like everyone else in every day life and its ups and downs. They did their best. I know, in their own way, that they thought the world of all three of us. We were seen as a family to keep up with on the surface. It was a strange duality, normality on one side and immense incongruence and emotional instability on the other.

Animal magic

Through all our challenges in communicating as a family we would find solace in a deep connection through our animals. When I was very young, we had a dog called Minnie, a budgerigar, a chinchilla and various types of guinea pigs. It taught us how to care for other beings.

My first treasure was a Shetland pony, diminutive in size, a piebald with attitude, full of character and like a very small carthorse. He was gorgeous. I first met him at the riding school my sister and I attended. I was very grateful for this opportunity. After a few lessons a new pony came to the stables. His name was Budgie and I fell in love with him straight away.

He was a troubled soul, wouldn't let many people ride him and was difficult to handle. I had no idea of this when I first sat on his back. He and I bonded instantly. I couldn't understand what all the fuss was about. Budgie was a dream to ride.

Over the coming months I really looked forward to our weekly lessons with Budgie. If he wasn't available it didn't seem or feel right to ride any other horse. We learned so much together and I know he understood and he made me laugh a lot. He was cheeky and had a face to match.

Dad's business was doing quite well and my sister was bought her first horse called Bambi, a lovely natured steady plodder. I was ever so slightly miffed that she had a horse and I didn't and felt I had done something very wrong. But after a few months continuing at riding school, Dad surprised me and bought Budgie. The school had to let him go as he wouldn't let anyone else ride him. I was in heaven. We kept the horses in a field that backed onto our garden and Dad had turned our own back garden into a paddock with a stable. It was quite a sight, the washing hanging up to dry with a horse in the background! My brother wasn't into horses. He was into music and played the horn in the local band and enjoyed mechanical things like cars. Like father, like son as they say.

We mucked out, fed, watered and groomed the horses. Mum was a fundamental part of all of this. My sister and I were in our element, we had so much fun, the bullying slowly reduced, as she had another focus. She and Mum still had complete control over my emotions though. Budgie was magic at gymkhanas. He would be like a slivery eel flowing through the bending poles and galloped like a rocket to get me to the finishing line many times. We won loads of rosettes. I laughed a lot, got nervous a lot and generally remember being really happy for the first time in my life.

We outgrew our horses. My sister was bought a beautiful white horse called Grey Lady and I was to have Bambi. Heartbreakingly Budgie was sold on. Gillian didn't like Lady for some reason and Bambi was too slow for me. As Mum was taking an interest in riding, she started to ride Bambi and it became evident that Lady and Gillian were not going to gel. So, I was very lucky that Lady came to me and Gillian had a new horse called Poppet, a feisty black gorgeous looking animal that was more suited to her character.

Lady was my soul mate, a beauty, so very loving and loyal. She would do anything for me. We would lie together in the field and she would lay her head on my lap when I felt sad and lonely. She was placid, kind and so very gentle. We galloped and trotted and walked through fields and common land, she was both responsive and responsible. We would dress up like cowboys and Indians and ride out for the day. I loved her so much. Lady would go to the ends of the earth for me, particularly in gymkhana competitions and we won lots of events together.

However, success breeds unwanted jealousy as I was soon to find out. My sister was jealous, and family friends who also had horses became jealous too. I have no idea why. They would do their best to knock Lady and I out of the competition. They were older and bigger than me. Gillian would tease and tell me I was useless and hated – not very pleasant, but at the time I believed her.

In amongst all the emotional ups and downs, Mum came into her creative element and made fancy dress costumes for us to wear as we competed in the shows during the summertime. It was so good and gave her a focus and purpose which she really enjoyed. It was lovely to see her engrossed in something other than herself and there were occasional glimpses of the mother who Dad fell in love with. Dad loved the competitions and would revel in us winning, although nothing was really good enough, not even winning. There would always be a, "but you should have done it this way." My brother was happy in his own way and came along to help out at the weekends. It was a fun time.

We lead busy lives. Mum was great and helped us muck out the stables and generally got involved with the animals. Good friends of my parents opened up a zoo not far from where we lived. Nigel and Jennifer were specialists in primate, big game and general animal care. Nigel worked for my Dad to earn some extra money, as he and his partner had a dream to open a zoo, where they could look after and give a home to what was then a rare breed of monkey.

Land was found in the grounds of a very old Elizabethan hotel in Surrey. Dad helped build these enormous wooden structures in and around the huge trees, so the monkeys could run free. As the zoo grew, we spent some of our spare time helping out. The three of us were in our element. The zoo grew to be home to a diversity of animals, gibbons, horses, birds, rabbits, geese and wonderful otters and very naughty mynah birds with whom you could have rather interesting conversations with!

I remember the first otter to arrive at the zoo. He was a rather special animal. His name was Midge and he starred in the film Ring of Bright Water. The book of the same name, written by Gavin Maxwell, was gifted to Nigel. My Mum looked after the otter enclosure. Playful, mischievous and incredibly dexterous, the otters where amazing to observe. Midge was incredibly loving and I am sure helped my Mum enormously. Other otters joined later as company for Midge. Animals were truly a saving grace in our family. They bought us together, gave enormous pleasure and were adored by us all.

I was about eight when a turning point came for me. Underlying our magical animal connection, I still hated school, my sister continued to be jealous and critical, Dad controlling and telling me what to do, how high to jump and when, Mum in and out of her depression and my brother being my brother. I felt like a piece of drift wood in an enormous ocean reflecting different moods like shades of blue.

The essence of water

It was a warm sunny day, our horsey friends had a small round tub-like pool in their garden and very often we would go over and play with their three children. Our parents would smoke, drink and talk, and sometimes we enjoyed a barbecue.

My Dad was an excellent swimmer, having learned the hard way with his mates, playing and fooling around in the gravel pits, not far from where he grew up during the Second World War. My Mother never had the opportunity to swim and was afraid of being out of her depth. I adored the feeling of being in water, but was terrified of letting go of the side of the pool.

One particular afternoon Mum and I were in the pool. She could stand up. It was too deep for me and I held on for dear life to the side of the pool. I couldn't touch the bottom, my legs flaying beneath me, I enjoyed the feeling of weightlessness.

Mum said, "Let go of the side."
Panic struck. "No, Mum. I'll sink."
"Go on, let go. You won't sink."
So I did. It was unusual for Mum to encourage me to do something she couldn't and I think it was because of that I let go. I cannot tell you how supportive I felt in this tub of water. I was floating, how amazing! I moved my arms and kicked my legs. It felt incredible. Then fear took over again, better grab hold of the side again, lest it may not last.

However, the moment did last and from letting go of the fear, in that one split moment, I never felt fear in water again. That split second in time, proved to be my saviour years later when I was caught in a tsunami. I started going to swimming lessons at school. How wonderful. Another sport to get lost in! The Headmaster spotted that I might have potential. He was part of a local swimming club and asked my Dad if he would bring me in for a trial. So, I did a trial in the small teaching pool at the local swimming baths, one length of each, doggy paddle with a bit of head up front crawl, back stroke and breaststroke. They must have seen something as I was signed up to join the club. This was such a far cry from the disaster of the ballet classes.

I continued to learn how to swim with the club and very quickly progressed to the big pool going from swimming widths to lengths. I was truly in my element. My best stroke at this time was backstroke, but as I soon mastered the breathing technique for front crawl this became my finest and strongest stroke. I learned how to swim butterfly which required an enormous amount of strength and technique and was later to be my favourite stroke to swim. The problem I had with my hair falling out abated and my hair started to grow in abundance. I ate like there was no tomorrow, as my body needed the energy to train. I became very healthy and fit indeed, no longer just a skinny kid.

I adored the training sessions. Once in the water, I was alone with my thoughts. It was so quiet underneath the water, just my breathing to listen too, completely at one with my physical body and mind. There were others in the training lane. We were all competing against one another, but I always knew when to push to hold a space and when to hold back from a space. I became known as the specialist in pacing. Even though I wasn't the fastest it was always, "Jane you go first, go on" and I would consciously drive or hold back the pace for everyone according to the timings set.

I enjoyed being in competitions to a degree, but I was too nervous and apparently not aggressive enough. Winning is important, I was told and I understood it to mean you must be better than anyone else. I didn't think so. To me, I really enjoyed the journey of training and getting into that 'zone' where no one else can go. Competition was an expectation to deliver an outcome and that took the essence away for me. If competition had been fun without expectation of an outcome, I am sure it would have been much more pleasurable. On the surface I enjoyed the thought of competing, but underneath I never felt good enough. Competitions left me feeling anxious about winning the next one. So, I much preferred the drills of training, where no one could touch me and I could excel.

In amongst swimming training I was still riding. Dad had made some very sturdy horse jumps – being an inventor, he never did anything by halves. He was known for fixing and repairing, making something work again, rather than having a throw away and buy another, kind of attitude. People would bring Dad their broken tools, cars, lawnmowers. You name it, Dad could fix it. He was a genius in that department.

On a particular summers' day disaster struck. I wasn't riding Lady, someone else was. I was sat on a sturdily made, very heavy thick pole that was held in place by the jump couplings. As normal, I was fidgeting, something I did very well. I always had loads of energy and was always being told to keep still. As usual I couldn't resist rocking backwards and forwards. Then it happened. Off popped the pole out of its coupling and away I went. I instinctively gripped the pole at the back of my knees as it rolled off backwards. I landed on the base of my neck and the pole subsequently crushed my tiny body, in a foetus shape, knees to my chest. Ouch, I couldn't move. The next few moments were a bit of a blur. In the haze, I remember being told that I was stupid for fidgeting. Well, of course, I was. Then concern became the order of the day as I was quiet. Tears streamed down my face and I was in deep pain. I felt helpless, like a rage doll and in shock. I could see Mum and Dad were deeply concerned.

I was taken to hospital and diagnosed as having cracked vertebrae in my mid back, a slipped disc and pulled ligaments in my lower back and sacrum. It could have been worse. Years later, I came to be very grateful to my parents, as after the initial diagnosis and treatment, they had the foresight to take me to an Osteopath. He worked wonders. I was in a lot of pain, but his gentleness helped my body heal. Of course, I couldn't ride for a while, but I could swim. Front crawl and back crawl were not painful, however butterfly was. It pulled on the ligaments around my lower back too much. I was not able to swim butterfly for two years after the accident. Swimming saved me in so many ways. The movement of my body with the support of water was incredibly healing. I still looked after Lady, how could I not? She was my soul mate and I was able to ride her again once the inflammation and pain had reduced.

I did so well in swimming that the horses became less and less apart of my daily routine. Training sessions in the pool became more frequent and took up most of my time outside of school. One day, Mum and Dad gave me the agonising choice between keeping and riding Lady or concentrating on swimming. I chose swimming. It was heart breaking and Lady was sold. It was a real wrench.

Swimming was bliss for me at that time and it was something I was a natural at. It seemed right, although I was heartbroken to let my beautiful white horse go. I never forgot my white Lady. She was my saviour and continues to be part of my life in thoughts and dreams. It was also another lesson to let go of things, for the best all round and allow for the blessings that can emerge from that letting go.

I was selected for swimming competitions more frequently and became the main stay of the senior team. Swimming meets were not entirely enjoyable for me, expectation and excitement was so evident in the air. Not only was I anxious and fearful, I seemed to pick up on so much anxiety and fear from those around me. I would calmly support my team mates, telling them to go for it and they will be alright, little did they know how I felt inside. The feeling was one of not wanting to be disappointing and wanting so much to please. I would love to win, however the thought losing was dreadful. So I would sabotage my thoughts and not think about winning, not really believing that I could anyway. The nerves were overwhelming.

What I really did enjoy was the feeling of diving into the water at the start, one minute you are sensing the atmosphere and buzz around you, then the next you are diving into the cool water, complete silence, only the sound of your own breathing and the movement of your body to contend with.

Then after the first few frenetic strokes, the rhythm takes over and it feels good for a while. Suddenly the mind kicks in and starts to plays tricks, a continuous internal chatter would follow. "How many lengths have I done? Was that length three?" Panic! I'd forgotten how many lengths I've done. "Let's look at the others and see where they are." Then I would lose my focus and my attention would switch to the other swimmers and I would forget my race. This was the complete opposite to training, where I always knew instinctively exactly how many lengths, at what pace I would be doing and where I was in the lane. The difference, I began to recognise, was that my instincts were always right, yet distorted and destructive thoughts could quite easily change a reality, so channelling the right thoughts were crucial. 'Focus on the feeling' became a mantra in later years.

There was one particular race where I really did notice how I unconsciously sabotaged a win . After a two year break from swimming butterfly, my back had healed really well and I had started to train in this stroke again. The extra front crawl training I had done in place of butterfly had built up stamina and strength, the transition to fly was technical rather than physical. Because of my stamina and strength, I quickly became good at fly.

My first ever butterfly race was 100 metres, four lengths of the pool. For some reason I was really looking forward to a fresh start, as I hadn't raced butterfly before, this could be my chance. The gun went off and I dived into the water. I felt good as I went out at a steady pace and by the end of the second length was in front by a mile. How exciting. Then I started to think, "Is this real? Can I really be this far out in front? I haven't raced this before, what if I can't make it to four lengths, what if I haven't paced myself?" Doubts crept in.

Half way down the fourth and last length I swallowed a bucketful of water and promptly stopped, gasping for air. I heard the crowd going, "Ah." I couldn't breathe and struggled to keep my head above the water as I clung onto the lane rope. The other girls gushed past me to the finish. I was in tears, devastated. I looked over to the line judge and other people on the poolside. I could see their mouths miming "Are you okay?" I shook my head, spluttering and coughing and did doggy paddle to the side of the pool to be helped out. I had never experienced suffocation before. I had choked in training, but this was extreme. It was very frightening not being able to breath. There was a tightness around my chest and nothing seemed real. It was like a dream. Slowly, my breathing returned to normal. I felt wretched and very sorry for myself. What a plonker! I had the race wrapped up. I hadn't run out of steam, I had just allowed the fear to overcome my exhilaration!

Doubts were not the only battles within me, there were battles at home too. My sister continued to be jealous of my success and would continue to tease me, but Mother had become jealous as well. I noticed she started playing up with Dad, being ill and saying things like, "You're not taking Jane swimming again are you?" Mum wanted him to herself. She had been very supportive of my training, but her visits to the training pool became less frequent. It must have been a battle for Dad.

Thanks to him, and despite the subtle manipulation and emotional blackmail going on at home, I attended all the training sessions and was never late. I think Mum was going through a really bad time and as swimming was becoming a serious way of life for me, she was less in control of me emotionally and possibly Dad too. I got the silent treatment from Mum. She pretended nothing was wrong, but I sensed that Dad was getting a hard time. It was normal for my sister to venomously attack me, but Mum was much more subtle.

There was lightness in amongst the greyness of life. My parents ran the swimming social club, to which they gave both time and money. Every year the committee would put together a gala float for the yearly procession through the streets of the town. With my Dads' connections, we had access a lorry which was to be 'dressed up' in the theme of the year as voted in by the committee members. One year we did The King and I from the film with Yul Bryner and my Mum made most of the costumes. She made a fantastic job of the detail, showing that she could do anything she wanted if she chose to do.

Mum and Dad, really enjoyed being part of something and making a difference, even though I knew they found being part of the social club sometimes stressful. Often, other people promised to do something then let them down, so they ended up doing most of the work to keep it all together.

One of the biggest events that was organised was an exchange trip with a French Swimming club. This was to be my first trip aboard, I was a little fearful of the trip. We were to stay with French families in Paris and take part in a friendly swimming competition. I was really nervous about staying with people I didn't know. Totally insecure, feeling like a fish out of water, being in a foreign country where they spoke very little English, I felt like I was three years old again. I didn't know what to say.

However, it opened my eyes to the realisation that there are other ways of doing things, other cultures to learn about. I particularly enjoyed the different ways to eat food and loved the morning meal, a huge bowl of chocolate drink which you would unceremoniously dunk tasty croissants into. That was most agreeable!

As we were there to compete, I swam quite well in the gala and came back with a gold and silver medal, and an experience I shall never forget. I had survived being completely out of my comfort zone. I took sea sickness tablets for the long journey on the coach and seemed to manage quite well. It was a trip full of fun with a great team spirit, a party atmosphere, singing and generally fooling around and laughing a lot.

As I got older and became, in a sense, more successful my sister started to be less abusive. Gillian was incredibly talented in her own way. A great artist, she could do anything she wanted to, but she resented any praise or offers of help. Independent and determined to do the opposite, that was her choice. Gillian had found another focus in boys.

On one occasion at school, for some reason I was being unfairly verbally attacked by one of the older girls from my sisters' year. She was a big bully. It had something to do with taking the mickey out of my hair which was bleached blond and like straw, from the hours I put in training in a pool of chlorine water. I was being chided as I looked different. My sister saw I was in trouble and came over. She could see I was upset and had tears in my eyes and stepped in and really stood up for me. After that moment I never had any problems with back chat from anyone else and continued to be part of the 'it girl crowd' from my own school year. For the first time, I felt I wasn't alone. I'll never forget that moment. My sister was later to become an ally of sorts in another event of my life. Maybe, she began to see me in a different light. I saw her in a different light and realised she was no different to me, she just reacted in a dissimilar way – her pain expressing itself through anger and control.

As we grew into our teenage years, swimming was my life. I had no idea about boys and actually wasn't interested. I had a great laugh with the guys in training and enjoyed their company, but training was my passion. Mum had made it very clear, that men are not to be trusted and they are only after one thing. Sex is dirty. Not that she ever explained about the birds and the bees to me, but I knew by the way she acted with Dad. So I never really got what the excitement was about. The girls at school started to constantly talk about boys. I just went along, not quite knowing what all the fuss was about.

I was not interested in boys but my sister, on the other hand, was a complete contrast she couldn't get enough of them. It must have been such an anxious time for my parents. She used to bring home young men and had a couple of serious relationships. I never really got involved. It was good to see her actually happy when she was with them. She was pleasant to me and even though I was often the butt of her jokes, I didn't mind at all.

The swimming continued. I got better and better as I swam in the counties and nationals. My life revolved around training. Early mornings and after school, in the summer holidays two weeks at the Crystal Palace swim camp. That was incredibly hard work and involved training with some of the top coaches around. The rest of my holidays were spent with swimming club pals. We used to go swimming in the river which is not advisable, but hey it was great fun. We were always in and out of some kind of water activity. As a family we would holiday in Ireland, Devon and Cornwall, and they always revolved around animals or water activities.

One year Dad treated us all to our first holiday abroad in Yugoslavia. It was our first time in an aeroplane. Strangely nervous and excited, I couldn't believe the feeling of flying. It was fantastic and I didn't get travel sick. When we arrived in Dubrovnik, I was struck by the beauty of the mountains, fresh air and the crystal clear sea and the warmth of the sunshine. I loved being in this climate. I felt really good. Dad and I used to swim out in the sea for what seemed like miles. In reality, it was probably only about four hundred metres. Mum would get worried and fret about how far we had gone. We would walk around the pristine town of Dubrovnik and marvel at the buildings and cleanliness of the streets. The people had a real pride in their surroundings. We generally had a great time there as a family and I got the bug to travel. I liked the feeling of freedom.

Slowly and inevitably my focus began to change. I was getting bored with swimming training. It really was getting serious and I was sacrificing a lot of growing up because of it. I was on the precipice of making it great or giving it all up. I needed more of a challenge if I was to continue. I had to make a choice.

Circumstances were soon to change everything for me forever which took away that choice.

OCEAN BLUE

"The Lehua blossom unfolds when the rains tread on it"
Hawaiian Proverb

Into despair

I needed a different challenge, swimming was becoming a chore. I was unsure what I was doing it for anymore and began to question what my purpose in life was. I started to get curious about boys. I was fifteen years old. My sister seemed adept in the art of boyfriend culture, and for the very first time she asked me if I wanted to go to the Saturday night disco, down at the local football club hall. My parents agreed that I could go. I was excited and nervous. I didn't know what to wear. I didn't do girly clothes things, not really. I wasn't into make-up or high heels and didn't see what all the fuss was about. It was swimming costumes and training gear for me, as that was what I felt comfortable in.

My sister helped me. She seemed quite keen to take me out and for the first time ever we were getting on. So, I chose a lovely dress, mainly black with a white collar and buttons down the front. It was pretty and it felt comfortable, smart and presentable. With Gillian's guidance, I put on some mascara and a little blusher and a smattering of lipstick on my lips. I was excited yet scared to death at the thought of not knowing anyone. "What if someone that I didn't know spoke to me? What did I say?"

It was a clear cool evening. The stars were bright in the sky. The football club was nearby our school. It had proper spectator stands, gravel car park and a single story building as the hub of the club. We arrived as the hall was filling up with people and sure enough I hardly knew anyone at all, just one or two familiar faces from school. The music was playing loudly, disco lights were flashing and there was a buzz in the air as people started dancing around. I stayed in the corner and observed for a while. My sister kept coming over to see if I was alright and eventually I plucked up the courage to have a little dance. We put our handbags on the floor and feeling a little self conscious danced around them – all was going well. I was actually enjoying myself. It was exhilarating, so much to learn and so many new faces. My face was beaming I just couldn't stop smiling.

I took myself off to the entrance to get some fresh air where a man, who was slightly familiar, stood smoking in the entrance. He started to talk to me. I wasn't interested at all, but he was insistent.

He said, "Come outside."

I said "No, why?"

"It's fresher outside," he said. Then he grabbed my hand and led me out of the entrance. I felt resistant and really not sure this was a good idea, and I hesitated, not understanding his intention.

My mind went into a spin. Somehow I was curious as to what he wanted and yet I sensed a great deal of fear in the pit of my belly. It was like I was two people. I tried to go back inside but he pulled me and grabbed me closer.

I said, "What are you doing?"

"Lets go down to the stands," he said.

"Why?" I said. "I want to go back in, leave me alone."

My mind still didn't connect that I was in a fearful position, as I had no idea what he wanted.

He must have sensed my confused indecision as being a signal and seized the opportunity. In one swift moment, he picked me up and threw me over his shoulder, like in a fireman's lift and started to walk down into the darkness. Fear took over, it must have been a comical sight, as he had me draped over his shoulder, my arms stretched out holding onto to dear life to a steel cold and slippery stand barrier, trying my best to resist being taken. I tried to scream at him, but it seemed to come out as a stifled restricted whisper. I had no chance, he was too strong. He hoofed me down to the stands, threw me onto the cold concrete ground, pinned me down and raped me.

I switched off, went somewhere else and disconnected – what was the point? A voice in my head said, "Just stay still Jane." I had no emotional feeling whatsoever, just the physical pain of the violation. None of it felt real. I don't remember screaming out loudly, I did remember kicking and punching. I did remember the pain and I did remember looking up to the heavens and switching off into the void.

Afterwards he walked back with me to the club house, like nothing had happened. I didn't say a word. I have no idea where he went, I had mud on my lovely dress and I ran bleary eyed into the ladies toilets, where my sister found me. I couldn't tell her what had happened as I didn't exactly understand it myself at the time. She could see something was wrong and through my sobs I asked her to promise me that she would not tell my parents that my dress was muddy and I was upset. I felt dirty and awful. Actually those words don't even describe how it felt. I was in shock and I couldn't make any sense of it at all.

How I got through the next couple of weeks I will never know. I was ill with horrendous headaches. Mum and Dad had no idea what had transpired. As far as I was aware my sister had kept her word. I felt disgusted, could not even describe the complete and utter destruction of myself. I was 15 years old. It wasn't even legal. My first ever experience with a man and it was horrific.

I eventually went back to school, continued to be shell shocked and stayed in my own little world. Nobody knew what had happened to me. I had learned that I didn't know how to express my deepest feelings a long time ago so I kept it all bottled up inside. Who could I tell anyway? I became depressed, wouldn't go training, and lost interest in everything. I felt completely closed to joyful activities. I shut myself in my bedroom and I cried myself to sleep at night, thinking what a bad person I was for letting this happen to me. I felt guilty, dirty and desperate. It was like I was stranded in the middle of a vast blue ocean, going down and down to its darkest depths, with no way out.

Mum and Dad showed concern, as I couldn't articulate what was really wrong they took me to the doctor as my headaches continued to get worse. The doctor diagnosed depression. Like mother, like daughter I thought. I was given some anti-depressants. I really didn't like the idea of taking tablets as I saw what they had done to my Mum but at this stage I had no energy or motivation to do anything else. It seemed what I least wanted was coming true. Hey presto, here I was feeling or not feeling as the case may be, so awful, exactly like my Mum. I really came to appreciate and understand how she must feel all the time, as I was feeling it now. Deep inside, I wanted to scream out. I didn't like taking the tablets. I took them for six months and wanted no more, as underlying in my unconscious was a sense of determination, hidden but coming to the surface through the depths of despair.

I grieved for my loss for many years. In the first three years I rebelled against my 'nice girl' character and started doing things that I would never dream of before. I really didn't care about myself. I stopped swimming and went out a lot to discos and clubs. I got my first taste of alcohol, which I didn't like, as it was the done thing, stayed out until the last minute I could and got into trouble with my parents. I became much more like my sister, acting up and generally not giving a damn. Proper teenage rebellion.

Far better for me to do things outside of myself, as I sure didn't like what was inside. I started to eat and eat and put on weight. This was not the Janie everyone knew. I never did anything bad, but I pushed my own boundaries many times and didn't care that I was acting completely out of character. Actually, I didn't really know who I was, not that I knew before as my identity was wrapped up in disciplined training regimes, but that was gone and the void went even deeper now. The emotional scars of this time would last and affect me for years after. For now, I buried it as best I could.

Everything in my life was a bit of a jumble after I left school. I went straight out to work, which gave me a focus of sorts. College and university wasn't the route to go in our family, going out to work was the done and respected thing. Dad believed that we should earn a living and learn through work, like he did. I started working as a shop assistant in a hosiery department of a well known department store. It was very boring, but a job and gave me a start in building confidence in interacting with people.

I never really knew what I wanted to do as a career apart from maybe teaching sports. But that was an impossibility as I wanted out from school and I couldn't see myself in continuing education. So, I half dreamt of a career as a make-up artist. My interest in art and colour coupled with an interest in the human body and skin, seemed the natural progression. This would have meant going to college and further education, neither of which were an option. So I decided to go a different route, a half way house if you like. After working as a shop assistant for a while, I was lucky enough to be given an opportunity to work for a well known and prestigious skin care company. I would become the youngest account manager they had. Initially I loved it. It gave me an identity and recognition that had been sadly missing since being a swimmer and an opportunity to learn a new skill. I really enjoyed this for a time. I met some great people at work and had lots of fun.

However, underneath the surface, deep inside, turmoil and confusion continued to rage and bubble up to the surface now and then. So the job began to lose its glitz and glamour image. The endless drudgery of the five day week, the same route into work, and the same work space became wearisome. The saving grace were my work colleagues, they made everything worthwhile. We laughed a lot and built up a strong bond, partners in crime in the world of skincare and cosmetics. All very girly stuff. The job taught me a lot about the surface essence of being female, the stuff that can make woman pretty and attractive. I had grown up only knowing the gritty gustiness of competition, discipline, exhilaration and the fun of active participation.

All the time my secret, hidden beneath the surface, gave rise to feelings of complete unworthiness. Utter dislike of myself and failure continued.

Escape to the light

One day a few of the girls at work invited me to join them on a back packing holiday to the Greek Islands. I was so excited, as it was an opportunity to have a break from work. This would be my second time travelling overseas by air. I remembered how I felt when we went on our first overseas holiday as a family. Freedom I thought. Mum and Dad were unsure, but eventually gave their blessing to go, I was eighteen. We were a right gaggle, all about the same age, two lovely Irish girls, who never stopped talking, my partner in crime at work, a kind of hippy fun loving type, another girl who was a friend of the Irish girls and me. I had the best time ever. We camped, swam in the sea, sunbathed and went out in the evening. We met so many people and for the first time in years, I felt free as a bird; no pressures or worries; a sense of clarity away from the clouds and confusion at home and so inside of me my spirits lifted for a short time. I loved the warm weather and blissful feeling of lying on the sand feeling the support of the earth beneath me. Greece was so charming. I fell in love with the islands and felt like I was home.

When I got back to work, I fell into a deep depression. All I wanted to do was to feel like I had on holiday in Greece. The islands beckoned. I was determined to go back, either on my own or with a friend. An inner strength, or stupidity, whichever way you wish to look at it!, drove me to make that happen. Reason and responsibility had gone out of the window and against everyone's advice, very blindly, three months later I handed in my notice at work and left a month later. I had made a decision to go for something and determination got me through. Still very shy and insecure inside, I packed a back pack. It was heavy and I could hardly lift it onto my back, maybe I thought I may never return! I left from Victoria coach station to take the trip down through Europe, France, Germany, the Swiss Alps and into Yugoslavia and then four days later arriving into Athens. What an adventure!

This wouldn't be the first time I would just take off, without any real thought for the future. It set me free with a deep knowing that it was the right thing to do in this moment of time. It was another step of discovery in my own university of life learning.

My legs were swollen from being on a coach for such a long time and I had to take sea sickness tablets to stop me from being sick. They knocked me out, so I slept a lot, without them I would have been very ill. I was sick once, on the Channel ferry crossing, but then so was everyone else. It was a long blurry journey, through some beautiful countryside. Noticeably the roads changed when we reached Yugoslavia, pot holed and in great disrepair. I was shocked to see women in black digging the roads, no sign of the men doing the heavy work. Such different roles were being played out in front of my eyes as cultures changed the further South and East I went.

The arrival in Athens was a bombardment to my senses. I got off the coach to sweltering heat in the middle of an unfamiliar noisy, smelly city. My intention was to get to the port of Piraeus as soon as possible and get the first ferry off the mainland to the islands. I didn't speak Greek and no one seemed to speak English. It was a nightmare. I couldn't even read the signs to get a bus. Panic struck. What on earth drove me to do this on my own? All sorts of thoughts and insecurities ran through my mind as it played tricks on me, I felt lost. I got the distinct impression the Greeks were being particularly unhelpful, maybe quite rightly because I didn't speak their language, but that didn't help me.

After a stressful couple of hours of walking towards the general direction of the port, not at all sure it was the right direction, I thankfully bumped in to a couple of girls who were English teachers taking there summer break, also heading the same way.

We teamed up and together we tracked down a taxi. It wasn't easy to get a cab, although there were loads around, they wouldn't automatically stop, you had to step out into the road to get them to stop for you, and even then it wasn't guaranteed they would take you. If the journey didn't suit them, tough luck! I remember years later, I went back on a nostalgic trip and was stuck on a Sunday evening in the port of Piraeus trying to get a taxi to the airport. They didn't like that trip to the airport, particularly on a Sunday. In the end a Greek businessman, also experiencing trouble bribed a driver into taking us both. It was the only way.

Anyway, it was great to have the familiarity of English speaking companions, but I decided I must learn some Greek. How stupid was I to think that everyone speaks English! This hadn't happened last time I was here, as we were on a tourist route. This time I wasn't. It taught me a lesson though!

We arrived at the port and the two girls invited me to travel with them and we ended up spending the first few days on the island of Paros. During the days I would enjoy my own company, meeting different people, in the evenings I would rejoin the girls and we would eat together and go for a drink afterwards.

Paros was special. It had a kind of gentle energy to it, bubbling along, not too elaborate and not too dowdy and sleepy. Rolling hills and beautiful white and golden sandy beaches dotted around the island. The port area was a mix of old and new tavernas, tourist shops and museums. It was busy during the day, but a sense of calm prevailed in the evening. Night clubs were few and far between as the tavernas provided most of the entertainment for both locals and tourists alike. I loved the island of Paros. It was quiet and beautiful and I felt incredibly safe, as I did whenever I travelled in Greece outside of Athens. I could swim and snorkel in the sea, walk over the rugged cliffs, relax, enjoy an ouzo in a taverna and watch the sunset before an evening meal all without fear. I met so many lovely fellow travellers, all with different stories to tell. Equally amazing, for the first time in my life I never felt sea sick on the ferries. What absolute bliss. I could finally enjoy the beauty and feeling of being on the open seas, without the fear of throwing up.

We travelled around visiting different islands. Next on the list was Mykonos which was very cosmopolitan. Pretty taverna's, jewellery shops and posh restaurants lined the harbour front and tiny brightly coloured fishing boats, bobbed up and down in the gentle swell of the ocean.

During the day Mykonos was a sleepy quaint and typical picturesque Greek island. Whitewashed buildings with blue painted shutters peppered the surrounding craggy hills and harbour face. Slightly more manicured gorgeous white sandy beaches set the scene for sun worshippers. Outside the restaurants that lined the harbour, octopus caught from early morning fishing trips, would be draped over canopy rods, drying in the dazzling heat of the day. Later they would be made into a delightful meze dish for evening dinner. After dark, quiet days transformed into bizarre night club raves, a colourful mix of extremes, people from all walks of life, mingling and partying there way into the early hours, almost a complete contrast to Paros.

Mykonos was like nothing I had experienced before! It had a reputation of attracting the rich and the famous, along with the obscure, bold and the beautiful. We didn't stay long, although extremely interesting, it held a different kind of 'on the edge' energy. We had seen enough.

Naxos, one of the larger islands, was our next port of call. Olive trees dotted over expansive rolling hills which you could see for miles. Much, much quieter and peaceful, here we camped and stayed for a week. Naxos was an island with an authentic lazy Greek way of life, the days literally melted into evenings and sleepy early nights. It was a place for complete restoration. The beaches were loosely peppered with the hard core sun lovers, nothing else much happened here. Very little excess energy was required in Naxos. Time to move on…

Ios beckoned. It was to be the next island on the trip. It was different from Paros, which was my favourite place so far, but I loved it here too, still unspoilt and untouched by mass tourism. The small harbour area was surrounded by steep hills. It was very pretty. We camped on the port side and would watch the big ferries come in and marvel at the imagery and perfect timing of docking these huge ships that towered above the tiny village. The draw bridge would lower and immediately a conglomeration of people, animals, cars and lorries would pour out onto the jetty with much noise, all in a matter of minutes. Then equally manically, those leaving the island would rush onto in all manner of ways, with no real order or control. Ready and waiting for the arriving unsuspecting back packers would be Greek landlords and ladies, converging and scrambling towards them, waving photos of their prized rooms available to let. A sense of tranquillity and calm would pervade the port area again once the ferries left and everyone had disappeared.

Everyday I would take the steep walk up into town, located on top of a mountain, at least it seemed like a mountain, probably just a big hill, through the white washed houses and into a very cute square. Ios town had a lovely feel to it. From the main square we'd go down the other side of the hill towards the beach on the green bus. The buses in Greece looked like something out of the fifties, hot and smelly with Greek music playing as the bus driver, red eyed from drinking too much Ouzo, would cheerfully charge the bus down the hill. It always amazed me how accidents were avoided. Particularly when the busses would be packed to overflowing with people hanging on for dear life, going down and around steep corners with sheer drops on one side, narrowly missing the odd goat, motor bike or car coming up the hill.

The ride was well worth it. At the end of the road a stunning long sandy beach stretched out in front, surrounded by huge mountains, an enclave of contrasting beauty. One end of the beach had a couple of lively tavernas, where music would play all day and delicious home cooked Greek food was served. Everything in Greece is about family. Everyone in the family would be a part of the business. It was all hands on deck and gave a wonderful friendly, warm, welcoming feeling. Farther along the beach you could fine peace, quiet and solitude. At the back of the beach, where sand became shrubbery and bushes, it was hotter. A crescendo of cicadas, sounding like hypnotic tribal music, would reverberate and bounce off the surrounding mountains and, at times, be almost deafening.

The sea was absolutely crystal clear. The days were hot and lazy. I had no energy to do much else except read, swim, sunbath and chat with different people. As the days' sun became softer and gentler we'd make our way back up to the town on the bus and walk down the other side of the hill back to the port and get ready for the evening. At sunset, we'd watch the skyline change its hue into a beautiful soft pinky orange whilst enjoying an early evening drink. We'd sit listening to the sounds of classical music in one of the bars in the port. Magical Ios is where I left the two girls. They were due to go back to the UK and I had another month or so to continue my travels. Santorini was next on my journey.

Santorini was a complete contrast to all the other islands. It was a land blown apart from the violent volcanic eruption over three thousand years before, which had actually resulted in the demise of the ancient Minoan civilisation. The port was deep below the town, a winding, treacherous road the only route up and down. Santorini town was a stunning splatter of white houses and shops seemingly clinging onto a dark rock face high above the port. Almost every building enjoyed an incredible view towards the volcano crater, the top of which was visible above the ocean, giving a dramatic backdrop to the gorgeous sunsets. Most of the beaches were of black volcanic sand and very hot!

I stayed on Santorini for a week enjoying watching the eclectic mix of people that came to marvel at this amazing barren place. I made the long trip back by boat to Paros, before heading across and up to Milos and Sifnos, two very little known Greek islands, where there were hardly any tourists, only two boats a week made the trip to service these islands.

Although fairly close to each other, they were of a completely different character. Milos was a geological heaven. Rolling hills intermingled with flat planes, red, black, green and white beaches, with a diversity of rock formations and colours. I hired a scooter and had a wonderful time discovering different unspoilt bays and seeking out the fauna and flora.

Sifnos in complete contrast was green and lush. Well, as lush as it could be in the summer heat. Grapevines grew everywhere. When I arrived I hopped on a bus as I didn't like the look of staying in the small port area. I wanted to discover the island, so I got off the bus just before a little town called Kastro, which was a dramatic little dwelling area built on a hillock. On the flat plains leading up to the town I went in search of somewhere to stay.

Walking a long the road on a blazing hot summer day, heavy back pack weighing me down, I saw this little sign saying, Room to Rent. I knocked on the door and a little old Greek woman, with deep furrowed lines on her face opened the door and ushered me in the room. It was ideal, cool, with a little patio area covered by vines, and a beautiful view out towards the little white town and through the valley on one side to the glistening ocean. Apart from the sounds of nature, it was incredibly quiet. Somehow, with my pidgin Greek and many hand gestations, we managed to negotiate a deal for me to stay. Who needs to speak the language when you have laughter, hands and loads of humility!

I stayed there for a good while as it was a perfect location, near to the small town, quiet and within easy reach of a fantastic place to swim. To reach it you had to climb down the mountain, on dry dusty rocks, a little treacherous for the unwary, but well worth the risk as the ocean was delightfully inviting. Deep blue in colour and so clear you could see different coloured fish and corals, deep, deep below. There were very few tourists on the island, but a small group of us would regularly hang out there, share lunch and stories, it was a very safe spot to swim and dive and it became a great meeting place.

The lazy days of summer were coming to an end and I had to think about getting back to the UK. My ticket was already booked or I could have stayed here forever. I had been travelling for just over two months

I had enjoyed watching the transformation between the hot blistering Greek summer, into a cooler, more unpredictable October and November season. Sunrise and sunset changed and a sense of calm started to permeate everyday life. The hoards of package holidaymakers had all but disappeared, only the serious travellers were left. The Greeks, with dark circles round their eyes began to close up their businesses for the winter hibernation time. The Greeks work hard. They have an eight month window of opportunity to make money for surviving through the winter. You could see tiredness in their faces. The seven day week, long days and very long nights take their toll. It doesn't stop there though in the winter time on the islands, the olives need to be picked. Families work together to reap the harvest – a real sense of community prevails. However the pace is slower without the pressures of serving thousands of demanding tourists, which gives space for the islanders and the land to breathe again.

I reflected back to when I first arrived, feeling lost and a little scared, yet excited and determined to step forth into the unknown. I remember building up the courage to walk off a ferry onto another new island, getting more confident in haggling for a room to stay in and trusting my inner instinct to hop on a bus to find somewhere to camp. This shy girl had come a long way and my confidence and sense of self had grown. All the confusions and insecurities that I experienced at home had disappeared. This was a truly healing time in a well supported environment.

I felt like Greece was my stomping ground. It was safe, familiar and, more importantly, the people were different. They didn't expect anything from you. I found them to be reasonably honest and respectful of me being a young woman travelling on her own. The Greeks were friendly, protective and extremely generous so I never felt compromised. Of course, I had to play the game and adapt, become flexible, but boundaries were respected and I felt a sense of safety that I had not experienced before.

I travelled to Greece at the end of 1970's and early 80's. It's a very different place now, since joining the European Union. The charm has become a little distorted. There are some areas that retain the magic, but like most places you need to go off the beaten track to find them.

Back with a bump

My flight back to the UK was at three am in the morning. I arrived at the airport in Athens many hours before time, as there was nowhere else I wanted to be in Athens during the night. The rooftop of the airport was a great place to sit on a warm night as you could see the stars clearly in the sky. I took the opportunity of laying down my sleeping bag with my pack under my head for a snooze. It was a long wait for my flight. I wasn't alone. There were a couple of other people doing the same thing.

An hour or so later, I woke suddenly, sat bolt upright, turned around and there was a man bending down, just about to take something out of my pack! I'm not sure if words came out, some did but they didn't sound like me, the voice was very deep. My reaction startled him and he scurried off. He looked just as shocked as me. My sixth sense had worked well! I turned round and realised I was completely alone on the roof top. It was like a bolt of lightning, fear and vulnerability filled my reality, I was back in my old world again, yet somehow I felt stronger.

I arrived back to a cold wintry UK. It was a shock. Unfriendly faces, rush, rush, rush, noise and pollution. It felt like I had travelled through a time warp. I quickly found another job and got back into a routine. I was feeling the blues and started to wonder what life was all about again. "It must be better than this surely? What am I missing? I feel I'm missing something?"

Life and my uncertainty continued. I had various jobs, none of which could hold my attention for long. Everything became predictable, could life be better than this? I began to think seriously about another career. I adored sports and anything physical, yet I had an active creative mind and I wondrered how could I combine the two. I was still a wreck emotionally and felt like I needed some structure and discipline like the swimming training used to give me. Perhaps that was the answer.

Army barmy

I discussed some ideas with my parents and had this fancy idea that the Army would be an option. I could become a physical training instructor, travel the world and be happy. Dad was thrilled. Off I went to join up. The Army career guys were very persuasive. I passed the entrance tests, but I was disappointed to be told that to become a physical training instructor you had to be a certain rank and the only way to get this was to join up and learn a trade, then transfer once you had gained a ranking.

They persuaded me to join as a Military Policewoman, and yes, it was indeed a persuasion, as I didn't see myself as a police person at all. They said the training was tough, physically and mentally and would cover almost all aspects of the Army as well as learning how to be a policewoman. Learning field craft, weapons, police work, chemical and biological warfare, the role of the Military Police during both wartime and peacetime and much more sounded very enticing. I was hooked. Although I couldn't quite see myself as a police woman I went for it anyhow. I had to wait twelve months to start as recruitment had been put on hold for that year.

One year later after walking into the Army careers office, I received my Army issue suitcase and off I went to basic training at the Women's Royal Army Corps. Discipline and fitness was the order of the day. I loved it, just what I needed. After six weeks of polishing brasses and boots, running and climbing, drills and shrills, we had our passing out parade, many parents attended, including mine. Mum and Dad were incredibly proud.

The very next day twelve of us were on a train on our way to the Royal Military Police training Centre in Chichester. On arrival at the station we were met by a stern looking, impeccably dressed Staff Sergeant, ordered to climb into the back of a four ton truck and off we trundled to the barracks. The journey, of course, made me feel sick. The feeling had returned, but I was so used to it that I just got on with it and held back the feelings of nausea. We were ordered or rather barked at to get out of the truck and run to our dormitory and instructed to change into physical training kit (shorts, t-shirt, trainers) and be ready in ten minutes to meet together again back at the truck.

All of us were excited, yet worried about the unknown. Again we trundled off in the four toner and after what seemed like an age in time, we stopped. We were briefed that we had forty five minutes to run and find our way back to barracks, no guidance, no direction, just off you go!

Adrenaline pumped through me. Only forty five minutes! Where were we? Which direction do we go? Using a combination of gut instinct and observation off we trotted. It took most of us about thirty five minutes to find our way. That was our first initiation into what was going to be a very tough course indeed. The guys in the career centre were right, it would be one of the toughest challenges in my life to date but the discipline of swimming training had prepared me well.

We had to run everywhere in the barracks, between lessons, parades and duties. You dare not walk. Someone was always watching and if you were caught walking an anonymous booming voice would come from nowhere to tell you to get your arse into gear! There were only twelve girls out of a company of about sixty and absolutely no concession was made for being female. This was not a problem for me as I was used to training with the best in swimming. I loved it. Others hated every moment and they didn't last. You could pick out the ones that wouldn't make it. Moaning and groaning, they generally could not adapt to a physically and mentally demanding regime. We were eventually left with just six girls.

My physical boundaries were blown out of the water. In fact, I had no boundaries. I was right up there with the fittest of the guys, never gave in and relished every moment of every challenge thrown at us. Those that struggled couldn't let go of their sense of self. The Instructors wanted to break you down. Anyone that fought it had an awful time and didn't last. With me there was nothing to break down in the first place! I could adapt, shift with the mood. I did everything to the maximum and beyond expectation. This was a personal journey of finding my boundaries. I didn't need them breaking down, I needed to find them.

Once I had proved that I tried my best, I was very much left alone. I strove to better myself, never having a problem with self-motivation and determination. The occasional reward was all I needed to spur me on. I even won best recruit a few times, much to the dislike and jealousy of some of the other girls. I loved to be the very best at everything I did. It gave me a sense of achievement, knowing that I couldn't have done any better. I was called names because I went the extra mile, but I didn't care anymore, that was their problem, not mine. I had made some really good friends who would stand by me no matter what, as I would them, they too were seriously committed.

However, the instructors tuned into my weak area, that of using my voice. It happened many times on the drill square and as I was always overshadowed by the height of those around me, I ended up hidden in the middle of the squad during drills. Being balled at by an aggressive sergeant, marching around a square, trying desperately to keep up with the long legs surrounding me, I found ridiculous and would often get the giggles. We were a slick team, but once I started the giggles it would become infectious and all our shoulders would heave up and down as we suppressed the laughter. We had big beaming smiles on our faces when we were turned away from the instructors, transforming into serious, focussed attention when we turned about and were going back towards them.

The instructors decided I needed a kick up the backside and that they would bully a voice out of me. They screamed at me to shout the commands. I felt foolish and silly as my voice was pathetic and weak in the beginning, which added to the giggles around me. "Louder!" they would scream. Slowly I found my voice. It gave me great confidence. I couldn't believe this sound was me! Was it me? I began to enjoy this feeling as it gave me a sense of power! I would think back and wish I had this skill when I was a child being bullied by my sister. She would not have treated me like she did if I could have shown this strength, nor would that man have violated me. I was so very grateful for this push. I cringed at the time but in the awkwardness of moments we often don't see the gifts we are given. It did me such a huge favour.

During a very hot summer, we were out on exercise wearing full combat kit, plus nuclear, biological, chemical (NBC) suits sweltering in the heat. We were skirmishing across a meadow in an attempt to come up unseen on a fictitious enemy camp. When we got to the other side of the meadow the exercise was stopped. The staff sergeant asked if he thought we'd done a good job, no one answered, we were all extremely knackered. He turned round and asked me if I thought we had done a good job. I knew we hadn't. It was atrocious and slack. If it had been a real scenario we would have all been killed. He asked again, agonisingly I said, "No, we didn't do a good job." I couldn't lie. I felt daggers in my back from a couple of the girls. He made us do it again! I was hated and I felt awful, but I put that to the back of my mind, got my head down and thankfully the girls also got on with it as they realised we needed to do this properly, otherwise we would have to do it again and again no matter what any of us said. This time we all made an effort and were let off the hook from doing more.

That night I'd been earmarked to be OC (officer commanding) for the night operation. I fretted inside, "Oh my God, I have no idea what I'm doing here." The girls hated me for speaking up earlier and making them do the exercise again. I could not mess up. The instructor was cool. He briefed me on what I needed to do and he would be shadowing me. We were to make our way to a valley a couple of miles away and there we would wait in ambush. The other instructors were to be the perpetrators. It was the dead of night and we'd been waiting for hours with no sign of the insurgents. Now into the early hours, everyone was tired and tetchy.

My mind started to play tricks. Things were moving and flitting through the bushes. Was it real or wasn't it? I really couldn't tell. I definitely saw someone or something, maybe it was a ghost! My mind was going crazy, the adrenaline started to rush through my body. So I came to the conclusion that it was the group that we had come to ambush and I sent the order to go in. Guns and shouts blazing, no one was there! It was funny at the time but not if it had been for real. I'd imagined I had seen people moving through the undergrowth and actually it was probably the wind moving trees and bushes around!

Anyhow, making light of it, all that pent up frustration was released and it got us out of the situation as we could have been there all night for nothing as it turned out. Making our way back, we realised the instructors, the insurgents, had fallen asleep! Our staff sergeant was really pissed off with his colleagues, so we ambushed them back at base instead. I was forgiven by my mates as we had a great time making a meal of the situation. It was certainly one to remember. Afterwards, it became a standing joke.

The classroom work was a challenge. We carried out security duties, night sentry duties so it was a killer when, the next day you'd be sat in class trying to stay awake, listening to lectures about the law and having to learn the Police Acts verbatim. The instructors were brutal. If they saw anyone showing signs of tiredness, they would scream at you to stand up on the desk. I saw a couple of colleagues fall off the desks as they fell asleep standing up, not a pretty sight. I enjoyed the detail of learning something new and once I got my mind into gear, applied myself totally and found it easy to learn the intricacies of a new subject. This was such a far cry from my school days where I struggled with normal lessons, here I learned quickly and passed exams with flying colours. I wasn't such a dunce after all it seemed!

Weapons' training was exhilarating and I managed to excel in this for some reason. I gained a high respect for the destructive power of weapons and a strong sense that none of this was to be taken lightly and one had to be totally responsible in their use. Where were the minds of men that had created such destructive things I would wonder.

My swimming skill stood me in good stead during my Army training days. I was selected to swim for the Army and I became part of a prestigious team. I passed out of training school, fit and strong with a new sense of confidence. The last few years since the trauma of the rape, had given me a whole new set of life skills, which I had been unconsciously driven to do by simply listening to my gut feeling and allowing myself to go with the flow.

MUDDY WATERS

"On the path to truth, lies never ending challenging choices, all are equal in the end"
Unknown

Rookie

On the surface everything seemed fine. I had a great start in the military, felt strong and confident to a degree and ready for anything.

With great anticipation and excitement we awaited our posting notification. A few weeks earlier we had been asked to supply our posting place of choice. Nothing was guaranteed they said, but they would do their best to send us to a place where we would like to go. I thought hard about my choice; somewhere warm with an opportunity to continue with my sports. Simple! Cyprus was my first choice, Hong Kong, because it was exotic, was my second. We were delivered our results by post. Initially I was disappointed. I had been fantasising about going to Cyprus, visions and feelings of being somewhere Greek and warm was very appealing. Anyhow, I was going to be sent to London, probably the last place I wanted to be, noisy, smelly and dangerous.

Our instructors did their best to make London sound like it was the most prestigious posting to be sent to. There were two of us going to London, one of whom was my friend and best buddy Katherine. That was a relief at least. London, we were told, was a great posting, high profile, good for the career, lots of 'special duties,' whatever that meant. "You have to be highly polished and professional at all times as the eyes of the world are on you," they said. "Don't let us down." It was greatly glamorised and seen to be one of the best postings.

I knew London as I lived about forty miles away and occasionally used to go up there during my wild days following the rape incident. I'd wander around Oxford Street and drink in the atmosphere and observe the latest trend setters, get my hair cut into the most modern wacky style and generally saw it as an interesting place to be. The noise, pollution and dirty underground air bothered me and although I enjoyed my trips, brief visits were enough.

At least I would be near to my parent's home. It was only an hour away by train and they were secretly relieved I think. I drove up to London Victoria in my very precious mini, which had been lovingly customised by my Brother and Dad. The mini had a kind of modesty about it, however, my mini had received a re-spray in a chocolate brown with a silver stripe on the bonnet, wide wheels and a special small leather covered steering wheel. It stood out from the rest, really cool, well I thought so anyway.

My underlying shyness and insecurity, forever bubbling under the surface, allowed me to retreat and hide away whenever I felt threatened. It was, in fact, a godsend sometimes. I could stay below the radar, keep my head down and graft. So it was that I nervously turned into the entrance of the London Royal Military Police HQ, driving up to big imposing blue wooden doors, with the familiar badge at the top, London District Provost Company – 'at your service Sir!' The outside of the building was nondescript, a typical old grey stoned building, with barred windows on the outside, which was nothing unusual in London, and with only one gateway in. You would never believe there was a whole community behind the closed doors. I pressed the button to announce myself and a very shiny sergeant popped out of the side door to greet me. I was told that I could drive inside and unload, then park my car in a special area outside of the complex. I was told it would be safe there until my parking permit had arrived.

As I drove into the courtyard, I was struck by the buzz of activity. People were smiling. They seemed almost human, so much friendlier after the sternness and discipline of the training centre. On the ground floor of the courtyard was the duty room, administration offices, workshops and the OC's office (Officer Commanding). The accommodation blocks were located on the second floor, split up with men on the right and women on the left. The third floor was our mess and television lounge area and on the top floor was the bar.

I was shown to my room, to be shared with my friend and colleague Katherine. It was simple and clean with a window looking out onto a small back street. The showers and washing areas were shared and we all took responsibility for keeping them clean, organised by a rota system.

Katherine and I had hit it off right from the start at training centre. She wasn't like the other girls. She just got on with things and kept herself to herself, a bit like me in a way. Tall and slim, almost waif like with short red brown hair and an elfin face, she struggled with the tough physical regime in training, but she made up for it with her attitude. There was a mutual respect for others' space in our room. We were in different platoons which meant that we had different duty shifts, so didn't see much of each other. Katherine went out with a guy in the Police force and her time off was spent with him. We'd make time every now and then to get together for a good old catch up as we had shared so many experiences since joining the Army.

I had two days off to get settled in before starting a shift pattern which consisted of one platoon day, two duty days, two nights and two days off. On the platoon days, we could be doing anything. One time we went and sat in the Old Bailey and watched a case unfold, another time visited a museum followed by a drink or two in the pub all in the name of team building and learning of course! These days were generally about bonding as a team, educational and normally very enjoyable.

I soon settled into the routine. Early morning OC run of about three miles at seven in the morning, four days a week and once a week a longer run of up to eight miles, always during the smelly, polluted rush hour traffic. Really healthy! All this was followed by early morning parade taken by the regimental sergeant major (RSM). The RSM's prerogative was to 'ball' us out for something that we were never quite sure of, ready to start the day. If you were on nights, you missed the melee of the morning ritual.

I remember one particular morning involving a very funny and utterly ridiculous scenario. For some reason the RSM had really got out of the wrong side of the bed. We diligently all stood in line for inspection and he 'lost it.' I've never seen anyone get so red and almost explode with rage. Apparently, we had slacked off and our appearance was terrible. He barked at us to go and get changed at once and then report back in five minutes wearing our best dress as well as our nuclear, biological and chemical masks with our red caps on top! Well you've never seen something so ludicrous!

This really tickled my sense of humour and many others too. We all thought he had gone completely barmy as he continued to bellow out obscenities. We quietly giggled and laughed as we ran upstairs to get changed and finally stood in line looking a right bunch of misfits in full regalia. We were faceless as we had our gas masks on, topped off with a shiny rimmed red cap. It felt like we were back at the training centre. That was the sort of bullshit that went on there, not in an operational unit where serious stuff happened!

Anyhow it was the RSM's place to order these things, we just obeyed orders and this particular order was cracking! The officer commanding decided to make an appearance, ever vigilant from his 'goldfish bowl' office, sensing this had gone on too far. He ordered the RSM to stand down the parade. We never really knew what happened, but the RSM didn't last much longer. All sorts of rumours abounded. I actually believe it wasn't anything sinister and he left for retirement, probably he had just had enough and was ready to leave.

Prestige

Our OC had also been posted from the RMP training centre at the same time as Katherine and I. He was very keen that I pursue swimming training as I had already represented the Army, when I was at training centre. It was seen to be good public relations for the RMP corp to have one of their own taking part in representing the Army in something sporty. I found a local baths and swimming club round the corner from our barracks and promptly joined the training groups. It was particularly challenging to make the training sessions as duties were first priority and no one really understood the commitment required to swim competitively. Luckily the daily runs helped with my general fitness and as this activity was part of a team, it felt good. The swimming training was a struggle. I had changed. I realised that those out in 'civvie street,' were different you see, they just didn't have the same sense of humour. As a result training was a chore. I was expected to represent the Army, so I had to do my best under the circumstances and hope that I had done enough.

The inter services competition was looming, one of the most important events in the forces sporting calendar, a friendly competition between the Army, Navy and Royal Air Force. The swimming team gathered in Catterick for three weeks of solid training and fine tuning before the competition. It was great fun. I was away from London and everyday duties! We stayed in very old, World War II type corrugated blocks of accommodation which were cold and damp. It didn't matter though as the sun was shining and we spent the days either land training, swimming or playing polo. In the evening we would play games on the guys and skirmish into their accommodation block and create havoc, doing silly things like taking their washing, moving stuff around or something else disruptive. They would then return the favour and create merry hell in our block after dark by sneaking in with water buckets and drenching everything. It was mostly innocent, and sometimes not, but always fun.

After the three weeks training, off we travelled down to Royal Air Force St. Athan in Wales. The fun and games stopped and now the rivalry was serious. For many years the Army women's team had never won the trophy. This year was different. We had a strong team and, after a battle, we won and held the cup high for the first time in twenty years. It was great to be part of a successful winning team.

I went back to my duties in London, such a contrast, a real kick in the teeth after such freedom. I was congratulated by the OC who thanked me muttering, "Well done, well done, hrrr hummm." He actually continued to do this for about a week or so afterwards. For everyone else it was a short lived moment and for me too as everyday life continued on with daily runs, special duties, night patrols and duty desk shifts.

Sleeping was a bother. As day turned into night the whole atmosphere would change outside on the streets becoming incredibly noisy. At the height of IRA bombing campaign, London was on constant alert. A never ending torment of sirens and cars screaming around the streets until the early hours, then a slight reprieve before it all started again. Right outside our accommodation block was a narrow back street, one of the hidden doorways lead to a women's refuge centre. From about eleven at night you would hear screaming and shouting and banging on the doors. The bag ladies would be coming in from the cold streets for somewhere to rest their heads for the night. They were just noisy about it. It meant that you would never really completely relax, always be on edge and hearing these women was somehow haunting and disturbing.

I really disliked the night desk duties as it was so boring. You had to stay put and be aware of where the patrols were, decipher the alarms, control the coming and goings of the entrance and man the phones. By two am it would normally quieten down and at three am in the dead of the night the eyes would droop, the head would start to nod and before you knew it your head would butt the desk which would wake you up with a start. This would continue until about five thirty in the morning where life inside the block and outside would slowly begin to wake up. Those early morning hours were normally torment. As we would only do two night shifts in a row, the body and mind never really got into the pattern and as it was so against the natural rhythm, it was much more disturbing to ones health.

During the day shifts there would be the normal frantic activity out on the streets, alarms would go off and the duty squad cars would leap into action from wherever they were, to investigate. I loved being out on patrol, especially in the middle of the summer. My perception of London started to change as we would visit certain people to build relationships with other authorities, organisations and police units. We were all here for a reason during this time of fragility and uncertainty, focussed on the same ends. I really began to appreciate the British mentality and ability to come together in times of strife. The amazing capacity for human compassion and survival instinct was all around us.

London became a special place, particularly on a warm balmy evening, thousands of people would move around like ants, an eclectic mix of cultures from all over the world would be wandering around the streets, some directionless, others with real conviction, rushing, pushing and sweating. There would be immense electricity in the air, with a potential for anything to happen. Oh what a joy! In contrast winter was completely different, dark, damp, depressed and secretive. Who knew what went on behind closed doors? We still had plenty of action. During the Northern Ireland troubles we were often on high alert and had to remain constantly vigilant, not ever completely relaxing, even in our secure unit.

Romance at last

I had been in London for about a year, new people came and went as the two yearly postings came around. London was also a base for the Close Protection (CP) team at that time, so when the guys weren't on active CP service they operated with us doing daily duties. I had just started seeing a man. I knew he liked me and I liked him, but he said he wasn't ready for a committed relationship, still hurting from his divorce. Our fledgling relationship was short lived as the reality of life in the forces kicked in. Frank was called to Kampala for a six month tour of duty. We promised to keep in touch with each other and off he went.

Whilst he was away, we wrote to each other and tried to keep the flame alive through letter writing. I came to realise the pressures of keeping up a long distance relationship. We lived in two completely different worlds. He was in a dangerous, insecure place without enjoying familiar comforts and nothing had changed for me. I was enjoying a secure known, comfortable existence with predictable daily barrack life. So our perception on life had changed. It's difficult to keep a connection and evolve the relationship when the understanding of experience is not physically shared, especially at the beginning of the relationship. When he left, we were in the first stages of a relationship, so there really wasn't a strong enough basis or history between us or knowledge of each other for it to survive. Each of us was faced with immediate priorities in different cultures. So the relationship became profoundly challenging at this stage.

Frank had been away for about three months. There was still a connection between us, albeit distant, but I enjoyed the thought of a potential partner and still remembered the times we had shared with a glow in my heart.

Gossip and news of a new arrival in the company announced the return of Peter. Peter had a reputation of being a great laugh and one of the good guys. He'd been in Heidelberg on a six month tour of CP duty.

I first met Peter in the television room where I'd gone into to find my friend. It was my day off. Peter was sat there watching something on the television and he was dressed in his sports kit as he'd been for a run. We started chatting and didn't stop talking for an hours. Duties intervened. There was something about him. He had a certain charisma. He was witty, intelligent and charming. I kept my distance as I was still thinking about Frank in Kampala and although it had been early days for us, I did still feel a sense of loyalty and connection to him.

Peter knew Frank and I told him about our friendship. This didn't make any difference to Peter, why would it? He saw my connection with Frank as just a friendship and nothing else. I realised my feeling was more than that. I thought a lot of Frank, but didn't know how to express this as he was so far away.

Time went by and Peter continued to court me. He made every effort to gain my attention, bought me flowers, took me out for meals, played music to me, sang to me, you name it, he did the whole job lot. I was flattered. I started to think less of Frank and convinced myself that our relationship wasn't a relationship, so why should I worry. Peter was here. He made all the right moves and I took it all in. My boundaries were grey. Missing Frank and getting all this attention from someone who was physically there all the time, was creating a dissonance inside of me. I felt like I was wading through muddy waters, with no sense of what was the right thing to do and curious to discover more about this man who showed me so much interest and attention. It was reminiscent of the lack of clarity that I had experienced when I was fifteen.

Peter was intense. He asked me to marry him and I said, "No." We'd only known each other for a short period of time yet inside I was completely excited and couldn't believe someone would want to marry me! For some reason it I didn't think he was really serious as it came across in a jovial way. He asked me again about a month later, I said no, again. Frank was on my mind and all I could see in Peter was that he flirted with all the girls and led them on. He continued to pursue me and did all the right things, but something was missing and I couldn't put my finger on it.

Finally, he took me out for a meal one evening and produced a small box and asked me to marry him again. He was persistent at least. Contained inside the box was a beautiful small solid silver rose broach which had been his grandmothers'. My heart melted and I was gone. "How romantic," I thought." He must really love me….." Warily I agreed. He wanted to get married very quickly which was odd. I did know that he was on the rebound from a long term relationship with a girl, who had finished with him, but I turned a blind eye and trusted he was over that as he'd seem so committed to me. My fragile ego loved the attention. No one had done anything like this for me before and being the romantic type, I felt swept away by the fantasy of a wedding and living happily every after!

So it was that I fell hook line and sinker into thinking I loved this guy. He couldn't do anything wrong. He loved me and I loved him. It was a fairy tale story. We would live in bliss and everything was going to be alright. However, every so often I would get this feeling, buried deep inside, of mistrust, which slowly would bubble up to the surface when I least expected it to. I had Frank on my mind. I had convinced myself that Frank wasn't that interested in me anymore. Blinded by a need to be loved, I had all I wanted on my doorstep. Frank seemed so far away now, but inside I felt awful and guilty about the whole situation. What a mess. How could I tell him? I thought I might wait until he got back from his tour, rather than write to him.

There was a lot of gossip about Peter and I, some for and some against. I was advised to be careful and not get involved with Peter. I didn't really understand why they would say that, perhaps they knew something I didn't. Maybe as these were my colleagues they were looking out for me, being the rookie in the team. I brushed it aside and could only go on how I was being treated by him at the time, which seemed genuine. We were like great buddies. He was really romantic and seemed to cherish me. Some also knew my connection with Frank had been quite strong before he left, maybe they knew something I didn't. I hadn't had any contact with Frank for about four weeks. Our last letters were friendly. I knew he was due back soon and I was worried and had butterflies in my stomach about his reaction to my news. I began to feel awful and wish I had written to him.

My worst fears were realised. Frank returned and we met up for a drink. Unbeknown to me Frank had a whole other agenda. He told me he wanted to get engaged and had gone and arranged for a party. He had kept it all a secret as he wanted to surprise me. I was devastated, as I had no idea he felt that way about me, the last I knew he didn't want commitment.

I felt really bad and a fraud as I then had to break the news about me and Peter. His face was a picture as the news slowly sank in. I cried my eyes out when we parted. I thought, "Oh my God, I have made a big mistake." But how could I back out now? Peter was waiting for me. What had I done? I should have trusted my small inner doubt. Complete and utter confusion took over in the next few days. Out of panic I had made a decision to be with Peter and therefore I would stick with it. I cut every other thought or feeling out as it was too much to think about how to get out of this all. It was too overwhelming. Deep down I knew Frank would have been a much better partner, however, I was bowled over with all the attention. I loved Peter, even though there were serious doubts about his integrity. I decided it was worth the risk. It also meant that I didn't rock the boat and create even more havoc, where families and others were concerned.

It was pretty challenging over the next month or so. Frank was going to be posted elsewhere which was a blessing in disguise for both of us. We avoided each other. It was the best way but very sad. I kept thinking how he must be feeling. Was he angry, sad, hurt, relieved? I would never know.

In hindsight, I should have waited and not committed to anything or anyone until I was absolutely sure about the integrity and strength of the relationship with either one of them. Hindsight is a wonderful thing!

Wedding calamity

Slowly, we started to plan the wedding. Peter and I planned to get married on the 17th December 1983. An ominous day as it turned out. I was excited, nervous and deeply worried about the prospect of everyone's eyes on me and being the centre of attention. It was a church wedding, although our family wasn't religious as such, Peter's family was.

A calamity of things happened that day. My mother and I fell out. I am not sure why to this day, only that she felt that I had not paid her much attention, so she blocked me out and got upset and took more valium to calm her nerves as it seemed I was the cause of her anxiety. I let it go and tried to focus on getting myself ready. I was completely on edge as my own insecurities kept floating to the surface. Dad had arranged for a couple of black Rolls Royce cars. Actually, they were funeral hearses on loan from one of his customers for the day! On the drive to our beautiful little country church, on a showery day in December Dad and I shared the short journey. Dad asked me if I was ready. I hesitated and said "Mmm, too late now" in a joking way, but with a sinking feeling inside. "Never mind." I thought, trying not to let on to my inner feeling of uneasiness. "Let's get this over and done with." I thought as I pushed aside any doubts.

As my Dad and I were just about to set off down the aisle, the heel of my shoe got stuck in the floor grating. Panic inside! It felt like I was being stopped in my tracks. I unstuck my shoe and walked on. After the ceremony, we flooded outside for the photographs. Fortunately, the rain miraculously stopped. However, and very funnily, the two black cars were manoeuvring in the tight courtyard and bumped into each other. Oops! Finally, half of our congregation that were due from London didn't turn up.

It was the day of the Harrods bombing. We heard the news at the reception. It was devastating. Our colleagues who had got stuck in London were recalled for duty. It was a blow for us both. Our friends and colleagues were in the middle of a disaster and we weren't there. Those not in the forces didn't understand. We carried on with the celebrations, very conscious of the trauma back at base. Sadly, a friend of my best friend Katherine was killed in the bombing. Years later I realised I had so many opportunities to wake up to the fact that I had a choice and needn't have gone through the heartache that followed. If I had listened to my gut feeling deep inside and taken things a lot slower, my life would have taken a very different route, but also it may have been a lot worse and not the best route in the long run.

Following our wedding we were due to spend Christmas with my parents. Peter had been called to go to Beirut on a six month posting and was due to leave early in the New Year. We had very little time together. Mother was still not talking to me and on Christmas day we had another bust up. It had been brewing. I cannot remember her words to this day, but they were hurtful. I had obviously done something to upset her, but didn't know what. I ran out of the kitchen in tears. Peter followed me into the bedroom. I was distraught. All the feelings of being an insecure little girl came flooding back. I was out of control and couldn't reason with what was going on inside. Mother must really hate me, or at least that's how I felt. Peter and I decided to go back to our unit and spend the remaining few days we had together there.

The next day I received a call from Dad at the barracks in London, something Dad would never normally do, to say Mum was sorry, she wasn't herself and would we come back. My heart melted, in spite of everything, I would never want to hurt my parents. We went back. The subject of the upset was avoided and not discussed. I was on edge with my Mother and so desperately wanted to be loved by her and I held it together for the sake of the precious time Peter and I had left.

Warzone

Peter left for Beirut on the 3rd of January. I felt bereft, worried and deeply concerned on many levels. I was worried for his safety, I was really going to miss him and I was concerned how we could hold our relationship together. He would be miles away, just like it was with Frank. How could it last? How do we communicate? Will he still love me and so it went on? The endless mind talk and insecurities were unbearable. I was deeply fragile where relationships were concerned.

During the first month, although missing Peter like crazy, I continued to function well at work. Then the bombshell, it was on all the news. Serious fighting had broken out and was in full flow in Beirut. Images of bomb attacks and people being hurt and maimed on the streets filled our screens. Where was Peter? The phone lines into the country were down, communication was impossible. I phoned the embassy. "No, Peter wasn't on duty and not at the embassy" I was told. Panic hit me.... "Oh my God...is he alive? " I wanted to know. I couldn't function. Tears were just beneath the surface all the time, underneath my exterior I was incredibly sensitive to everything and on the very edge.

As no news from the Ministry of Defence was forthcoming, after my shift I would spend my time in the public call box outside in the street, trying to get a line into the country to the place where Peter was staying, without avail. My OC called me in to his office one day and like a father figure asked how I was doing. After telling him that Peter was missing, he told me not to worry, he would use his contacts to see where Peter was and in the meantime I was to be his personal driver so he could keep an 'eye on me.' This meant no shift work for a while which really helped as shift work was not good for sleep patterns and I was tired from worrying.

Three weeks later I had a call from the Embassy in Beirut. It was one of my days off and I was in my room. I was called down to the office. Peter was on the other end of the phone. At last he was alive and safe. He'd been caught up in a battle outside of the embassy and with the lines down couldn't make contact, mobile phones did not in exist in those days. His apartment had become a refuge in the middle of a battle field and there was no escape. What relief. Really, an absolute relief. My whole body relaxed. I was exhausted and shed a bucket load of tears of relief back in my room.

We spoke nearly everyday after that for a while. I would go to the public call box and we would arrange a time to call. Sometimes it would take up to two hours to get a line in, but we persevered.

Those six months were the longest of my life. The last two months or so, the calls reduced to once or twice a week. Things had settled down out there and he had made some local friends and I sensed a change in him. He didn't seem too interested and I felt the calls were a chore, a function rather than a joy. My old deep feelings of insecurity began to raise its ugly head again. My mind started to wonder what he was hiding, what he was up to. This didn't seem right. Little did I realise that he must have been suffering from what he had seen and been involved with, but I was also suffering.

When he got back, we stayed in our single accommodations in the unit, knowing that we would be posted in the next three months. It really wasn't worth us getting settled in married quarters for that short time. Life and duties continued and we managed to share some special moments during the rare times we could be together. I couldn't wait to get posted so we could set up a home at last.

In the meantime, I was chosen to go to India on a trip with the then Prime Minister, Margaret Thatcher, and her delegation to the Commonwealth Heads of Government meeting in New Delhi. What a privilege, three weeks to an unknown country and a chance to experience a different world. I was very excited. The whole trip opened up a new world. The past eight months had been horrendous. This was such a blessing in disguise. Someone's looking after me I thought.

Contrast

Arriving in India was a bombardment of the senses, colourful, vibrant, noisy, smelly and beautiful. There was starkness, a complete division of wealth. On the one hand, great buildings making grand statements, and on the other, complete poverty and depravation. It was extreme. People on the streets in the heat and dust were living out their lives in the gutter, scrabbling for any food or any item that would make money. Barbers went about their business on the roadside, out in the open, leaving the debris of shaving, hair cuttings and skin in the gutter where the children played.

The sacred river of the Ganges was equally enthralling, a vast expanse with a shoreline of women washing laundry and lines of clothes hung out to dry, draped between the iron pillars on the great bridges. People and animals bathed in this dirty muddy grey channel of water. It was raw survival on hand for all to see, if you chose to. It would have been easy to hide away in opulence and shut this other reality out of sight.

On the flip side, huge beautiful, clean buildings behind walls and big gates hid a completely different reality. I am grateful that I experienced, with all my senses, this incredible landscape of humanity and stayed open to receive the wonders and beauty in all things. From an outsiders point of view, life seemed confused, faces sad, terrible, raw survival on the edge. However, in amongst the throng, life flowed seamlessly on the streets. No solid pattern just complexity and contrast gracefully married together.

Happily, I was with some great colleagues and on off duty times we were allowed to attend the delegation events and trips out. That's how I ended up at the Taj Mahal in all its glory. How fitting that I should visit the Taj Mahal, one of the seven wonders of the world, built out of love. A place where the epitome of love emanated throughout this beautiful enormous monument. It took twenty two years of painstaking work by twenty two thousand workers to construct. An amazing feat of determination to bring a vision into a solid reality.

I came back from India, tired, yet somehow revitalised inside. A real spiritual awakening emerging from what I had experienced. When I returned, plans were being made to get Peter and I posted together. I was due to go to Northern Ireland, Peter was due to go to Germany. My OC put in a request for me to be able to join Peter in Germany. I still wanted to transfer to the physical training corps, as I had a ranking now but this wasn't the time, marriage was more important than my career and we had a lot of reconnecting to do.

Peter came home from Beirut a different man and no wonder. What he had been through would change anyone. Like all our serving soldiers, the enormity of the experiences that he went through day in day out and the complexities of the thoughts and emotions that he buried because they were too painful to live were difficult to understand. For a while he was introverted and secretive. At the time, I couldn't get my head around it. Where was this romantic, charming, open man that I had married? I was still very young and inexperienced in relationships. I also had suffered my own emotional roller coaster and the past six months had taken its toll. It all felt well, flat. Apart from the trauma he had experienced, there was something else that I couldn't put my finger on, something lost or maybe it wasn't there in the beginning. Was it in me or him?

We moved to Germany. He joined the CP team and I started shift work and police duties. It was much more laid back there, less intense than London and not so high profile. We lived in a big apartment about eight miles from our unit. Initially we didn't have a car, so we bought a couple of push bikes. It was great. It kept us fit and it was an easy ride in and out of work. Germany was light relief from the intensity of life back in the UK.

The first few months, everything was new for both of us. We enjoyed a good life in the times before the Euro. We ate out a lot and enjoyed strolling into our local town and sampling the many different pubs and restaurants on offer. Life seemed pretty good. Peter was happier and I was happier as I could throw myself into physical activities. I enjoyed the public sports facilities, an athletic track, trim trails through the nearby woods and a great swimming pool. It was a far cry from ours in the UK. We made friends with other married couples and exchanged social visits to each others houses. I enjoyed cooking and making a home, yes, life was good.

Whilst he was at home base, Peter worked a regular nine to five whilst I continued with shift work. He liked a drink, drowning his sorrows and sometimes used to stay out with his colleagues after work. At first, I accepted this, however, as it became a bit of a habit, I started to question his motives. As my insecurities started to surface, I found it difficult to express how it made me feel. I expected a call if he was going to be late, so I didn't worry and secondly, why did he feel the need to be away from me. My neediness and emptiness started to become a problem in our marriage. His disconnection and wanting to live a single life, being with the 'lads', added to and exacerbated the problem and I began to feel even more confused, isolated and lost again.

We'd been in Germany for about a year and our marriage had become dysfunctional, to say the least. I was resentful, coupled with the fact that I felt he wasn't listening, he was distant and not interested. At this time, I found out that my Dad had throat cancer. I felt trapped, worried and anxious. I was stuck in a strange land, in a marriage that wasn't entirely going to plan and wanting to be with my parents. I knew on one level Dad would be coping in his own way. Mum on the other hand would not be. A real tug of responsibility raged inside. Very similar to the feeling of when Peter was in Beirut, when I didn't know if he was alive or dead. Worry and anxiousness were forever beneath the surface.

I was on the edge emotionally, getting more and more insecure with Peter. I was trying to fathom if my mother was telling me the truth, or if her truth was based on her own stuff. Mum, bless her, would relate anything to get her own needs met. I would get one story from Mum, who told me how bad Dad is and how he was treating her and another from Dad, who would tell me that he was doing okay and not to worry. I had to trust what he said in the end as I was getting sick with worry. I wasn't there to see every day. I would get to see the truth when I went back on leave to find out for myself and actually it turned out that my gut feeling was right. Dad was managing his illness with a logical mind and seemed to be doing fine under the circumstances, whereas Mum was an emotional wreck. She couldn't cope. Dad wasn't there to hold her together and it scared her. The thought that Dad may not always be around created a huge amount of anxiety in her.

Dad had to have treatment for the cancer. It was a horrible treatment, an aggressive bout of radiotherapy, which effectively microwaved the throat area. Dad always loved to talk and be social, now he couldn't do anything except sit and listen as his vocal cords had been damaged by the treatment. It must have been incredibly difficult for him. But he was determined to meet and gather socially with his friends down the pub, even though he couldn't speak he could listen and use a pen and paper to communicate. It took over a year of uncertainty, to get the all clear from the Doctors. Luckily the cancer had been caught in time and it was restricted to the larynx. The treatment had gone well. Dad had been left with some horrible side effects following the treatment, but he was alive and eventually got his voice back.

Whilst all this was happening, I felt like I needed some stability at work. So, I applied for a position to work in the headquarters which would mean no shift work. I talked it over with Peter and we agreed it might help our relationship by having a regular pattern. I got the job and started to work a regular nine to five pattern, the same as him. This way we could spend more time together. I really enjoyed the regular hours and I expected things to change in our marriage, but they got worse. My insecurities were rife. He continued in his same pattern, drinking and staying out and I became this person that I didn't recognise, jealous, moaning, critical and angry. Who was I? I didn't know anymore and didn't know how to communicate my feelings as, when I did, they were dismissed as being invalid.

In the meantime, Dad was recovering well. He had a positive attitude. The blessing as well as getting better, was that he had stopped smoking. What a relief. Mum continued to smoke until she herself had a very bad bout of bronchitis a couple of years later and she stopped immediately after that. After so many years, it took serious illness to make my parents stop smoking. In their day and age it was such an accepted thing to do. It's ironic, that they finally understood what it was like for us as children because they came to dislike the smell of smoke themselves!

Peter continued to drink and not come home straight away after work, which was fine when he called to let me know, but not fine when he disrespected me and didn't tell me. I would worry about what he was up to and had no trust in him anymore. In fact, it was trust that was missing in the first place when I first met him, that niggling doubt inside. On the surface we kept up the pretence that everything was well in our world. We went to the mess events together and would have friends round for dinner. But I became suspicious of everything he did, not a very pleasant way to be with someone. He went away for anything up to four weeks on jobs, during his absence I found myself enjoying my space and thrived on the activities I did. It didn't stop me being suspicious of his antics whilst he was away. The strange thing is I began to resent him coming back. It upset the calm and easy routine in my own little world.

Normally, after he was back for a week, the general pattern of life would settle down and it became easier again as we adjusted ourselves around each other. I would do the wifely things, like sending his jackets off to the dry cleaners and twice, on two separate occasions, I found a girls name and hotel number or telephone number on bits of paper inside his pockets. My stomach would turn over and a deep sinking feeling would prevail. My immediate response was to hit out and accuse him straight away. The first time I asked him who this was he made up some feeble excuse, well I thought it was feeble, and all that did was confirm that my feelings were right, that he was playing around. That mistrustful feeling I recognised right in the beginning was playing itself out. What had I created?

He didn't deny anything and he said it was all innocent. Yeah right! I thought I had no choice but to believe him. The second time just blew any belief I may have had in him out of the water and I never trusted him again. Even more devastating was how he would ignore me at social events. No wonder, as I had become over- bearingly jealous and very sensitive to anything at this stage. I felt stuck and trapped and at that time couldn't see a clear way forward. The gap between my feelings and what was staring me in the face simply wasn't acceptable, yet I was allowing it to happen. I didn't know who or what I was anymore.

I remember once we went to a black tie evening do in the mess. A new officer had arrived in our unit. Peter, ever the social butterfly, would make a bee line for his wife. He would charm and romance and use his skill to chat and win her over. Sounds silly, I know, but he asked her for the first dance. He had ignored me all night and I felt further humiliated. I was his wife, why didn't he ask me to dance? Surely I should be the first one? A couple of people had noticed that I had withdrawn and came over to see if I was alright. On the surface I was fine; underneath I was in a rage!

On the way home, cold silence, I couldn't speak to him. Eventually, when I did, the words tumbled angrily out, I felt wretched. The evidence of his infidelity past and present, confirmed all of my fears from the moment I met him. His actions were further confirmed a year or so later, when we had left the forces, in yet another blatant incident of infidelity. The hesitancy that I felt and noticing something was a bit amiss had been there right from the start. My gut feeling had yet again been right, even though it was at a time when I was confused and really didn't know who I was, my sense of hesitancy was absolutely spot on. It was ever so subtle and another sign that I could trust my instinct. It just needed to get a little stronger.

At this horrible time, I felt so low. I really could not see a way out. I could not be with someone who would be unfaithful to me and not be honest about their feelings towards me, or could I? I would switch backwards and forwards between my thoughts and feelings. What was the alternative? I had given my all to this man and I felt guilty, knowing that I had known it wasn't right in the beginning. Yet I still carried on. This scenario was making me unhappy and I prayed for a way out.

Eventually on one of his long trips away, I got myself together and focussed on all the good times we enjoyed, the laughter and the pleasure we had in building a home of sorts and the friends we had made and the moments of romantic love that we had shared, albeit in the beginning. Funny though, that I must have been treating him with such disdain, but neither one of us wanted to let go of it. So we were stuck. Neither one of us wanting or knowing how to get out of this mess.

In an effort to salvage our deteriorating relationship, we talked about different options. I was due a posting to Northern Ireland, which meant we wouldn't be together this time. I also wanted to pursue my career as a physical training instructor which meant a move to the UK. However, he promised that he would change his behaviour and I suggested that I would come out of the army and be a wife at home for a while. He liked that idea. He would then hand in his notice later and we would become 'civvies', buy a home in the UK and live happily every after. My own plans to progress in the forces became a second priority and, out of my insecurity and feelings of worthlessness, I put my marriage first. Initially, this turned out to be a mistake. However, a year or so later, it became another blessing in disguise and my path lead me to receive some deep needed healing.

It was a hard decision to leave the Forces. It had been a home for me, familiar with wonderful camaraderie and great experiences. I had done well and would have continued to do so. I guess I was running away and taking the easy option. Emotionally exhausted, I couldn't face going through a split and having to keep a brave face on everything at work, where everyone would know. It was easier to try and work on the relationship and not have the responsibility of my career as well. As it turned out, it was a way out that led the way to me opening up to a different kind of awareness and eventually led us both to release ourselves from our torment.

Reprieve

So, six months later I left the Army and found a part time job working as a practice manager for a surgery for Army dependants, still based in Germany. I worked for a brilliant, highly intelligent doctor. He was different. He had come into practise late in life, with a background specialism in psychiatry, how wonderfully apt! Everyone loved him. He would be ridiculed for his 'strange and wacky ways' but for me he was a special person. His surgery would always run over time. He believed in spending time listening to patients rather than handing out a pill. I saw many people wait for hours to see him, without complaint.

I would make him a special brew of herbal tea and organise anything practical, as even the simplest of arrangements would be a challenge for him. He was incredibly untidy and disorganised. Every morning he would cycle into work, come flying into the surgery, collar half in half out, cycle clips on one leg and not the other and hair dishevelled. I basically put him together, tidied up after him, and ensured the right patient notes were in the right record sleeve, as he would very often get them mixed up!

He was truly brilliant. He taught me how to meditate, how to quiet my mind by sitting watching a candle. At first I felt silly and self conscious, but there was something calming and magical about watching a candle. I then found myself experiencing traumatic nightmares. I would wake in a cold sweat after seeing frightening hallucinations. It would wake Peter and he would have to calm me down and tell me everything was alright. He was good like that. They continued until I left to return to the UK. I forgot about them until years later.

The doctor helped me a lot, without me being aware of it. Years later I really thanked him in my prayers for showing me a different way. He somehow sensed my inner anguish, never said anything, but he knew. When I left he gave me an owl that he had made and painted, it was a very special gift. I still treasure it to this day.

And so it came to be, that Peter completed his twelve years Army service and we left Germany for good to start a new life in the UK. We bought a new house near to Bath in the beautiful South West of England and it was an opportunity for us both to create something together for the first time. However, it became increasingly apparent that Peter wasn't adapting well to civilian life. He missed the thrill and camaraderie of being in the forces in a tight knit unit and hated having the responsibility of mortgages and paying bills.

Our time together seemed false. I still didn't trust him and this underpinned any deep intimacy available to us. One day he had a call from a mate of his, ex forces, who said there was a job going overseas. Peter came alive again. I didn't care anymore and was thankful that he would be doing something he enjoyed. I was supporting us by paying the mortgage and all the bills so it was a great relief to know that there would be a second income coming in. I was doing a job that I hated and getting ill over it and this would take the pressure off me.

The job was in Washington DC, USA. I wasn't allowed to go with him for the first six months, as he said that he wanted to settle in and see how it went. With a sense of relief and sadness I let it all go and off he went. The truth was, that I could have joined him very quickly, he had a wonderful apartment and the other guys in the team had their wives with them. But it was the same scenario, the wife at home allowed him to be free and enjoy the single life again, it was all so convenient. He knew I would accept this as I had done before, this time though there wasn't the security of it being the norm as we weren't in the forces. I did have a choice now and I was ready to make a change. The moment he left, I felt free. Isn't that awful!? I really did feel happy.

Peter called me a lot in the beginning and every time kept on promising me that I would join him soon. This was a long term contract so there was no reason not too. It was nine months later when he eventually invited me over for Christmas. I really wasn't interested in seeing him. I was completely shut down to him. Peter being away allowed me the opportunity to train as an instructor in various disciplines. I didn't quite make it through the Army channels, as I had focussed on my marriage, but managed to do it now. I began to find myself again. I enjoyed my simple life, loved teaching swimming and other sports, watching kids and adults achieve something they didn't think possible. It was so rewarding. So, that major decision of leaving my forces career behind had actually lead me to a space where I could pursue my passion and get some strength, calm and serenity back into my life.

Christmas loomed and off I went to see him, nervous as it had been nine months since we were last together and I knew I had changed since the last time we had seen each other. He was the old charming self as he showed me around his apartment. I became immediately suspicious again when I saw it. I couldn't understand why I hadn't been before. There was plenty of room and would have been a great place for me to be as well and it wasn't as if money was the problem. Anyhow, I didn't care, it was so evident to me that I felt nothing for him anymore. He didn't seem to think that there was anything wrong, everything was fine in his eyes. I was incredulous. That's how we left it. I came back after Christmas, back into my life at home and he went back to his life, still promising me that I would be over soon. I had stopped listening. It was all talk and no action as normal. I had a new life and I wasn't going to let anyone interfere with that, married or not.

The next three months I became a little insecure and I avoided deep discussions with Peter. He sensed something was wrong and immediately wanted me to go out and stay with him. I told him I couldn't, my job was important to me. I started to get real, this wasn't a marriage and if I could survive on my own, why be married? I kept thinking backwards and forwards. "What was the benefit of us staying together?" Nothing actually. He was earning a lot of money, but it was for his life as I couldn't see how we would work, money or not. I decided to ask him for a divorce and as we weren't together had to do this over the phone. It set him off in a spin. He couldn't see why. He thought I was happy, invited me over to stay for good straight away, I could have come sooner and so it went on, all a load of bullshit.

I stuck to my guns and I started proceedings. He didn't contest anything and we mutually agreed to split everything down the middle. I really think he was secretly relieved. I hadn't exactly been a trusting, loving wife in his eyes and he certainly hadn't been able to meet my needs either. It was sad. Apart from anything else, we were still friends and I believe that's what kept us linked together for so long.

He came back on a summer's day in June to collect his belongings and take what he needed from the house. I acted terribly. There was so much pent up unexpressed anger that came up. I let loose. He just stood there shocked at my reaction to him. He said he was sorry to have hurt me and left. That was the last time I saw him. We had agreed that we wouldn't want to see each other again as strangely, it would have been too painful for both of us. We had one other contact about six months later. Peter had returned to the UK and needed some insurance details from me. It was a curt and quick conversation and that was it. Nearly six years of extreme emotional ups and downs was over.

I was later to be able to reflect back on my part in all of this, the rape and lack of self worth had left an enormous legacy in so many ways. Yet all through this, I did have an innate intuitive sense that I knew things weren't right from the start but I chose to go ahead with it anyway.

During the later stages of the divorce, I had struck up a friendship with a fellow instructor. He was steady, easy going and available. We shared a common ground in what we did. We became good friends and he helped me realise there could be life after marriage and I could be attractive to other men.

AWAKENING SPRINGS

"The truth is that our finest moments are most likely to occur when we are feeling deeply uncomfortable, unhappy, or unfulfilled. For it is only in such moments, propelled by our discomfort, that we are likely to step out of our ruts and start searching for different ways or truer answers."
M. Scott Peck

Emerging truth

Here I was living in the West country UK, in a beautiful location. My house was south facing on the edge of a valley and the views over the surrounding countryside were truly amazing. The sun shone into the lounge area from the East in the morning. It was stunning.

The new man in my life was completely different to Peter. I felt I trusted him from the moment I met him, no doubt about it. It was the first time I had ever felt this way about someone. His name was Steve and he was solid, respectful and honest. He was a few inches taller than me, had short dark hair, a friendly face, good sense of humour and, as an ex gymnast, had a fit body. We shared a common interest in teaching and sports. Steve practised karate. His mentor and teacher was from the old school and his teaching was all about respect, discipline and the more spiritual aspect of practise. His lessons were based on authentic traditions. I became interested in this style of martial art and joined the club. I felt like I was waking up to another reality. I relished the hard training sessions, the discipline of mind and body and the peaceful centeredness of calm during the meditations. Like Steve, I diligently continued training in the disciplines of the forms at home and with his help worked my way through the rankings. It seemed life was coming together for me again.

I really felt good about myself. This was my time. I was doing a job I loved, had a man that I trusted and a common activity that we shared. We were happy and content and enjoyed going to training sessions together, competitions and socialising with friends. I was still teaching sports and gradually moved into management. My career was going well. During the next three years of sharing a life together, I really began to find my feet again. I didn't have to worry about what Steve was doing as he was dependable and supportive in so many ways, sometimes a little possessive but a complete contrast to Peter. I found it interesting that I had met a complete opposite to my ex husband. Here was an opportunity to experience trust in a relationship, something that was new to me, but very welcome. I began to realise that my inner feelings were always right and my experiences so far had proved that. So, I became more settled and trusting and as those feelings strengthened, something ugly inside of me started to re-emerge, like an awakening spring. I was nearing my thirtieth birthday.

Leading up to my birthday year, Steve wanted more of a commitment. In his eyes that meant a share in my house. He placed value on material things. In my eyes commitment meant engagement and marriage. I had bought my husbands' share of the house from our divorce, so it was completely in my name. It was a strange time. I felt a strong need for love and affection and couldn't bear the thought of losing Steve by saying that it just didn't feel right. Out of a misplaced sense of love, I duly signed over half of my house to Steve - crazy eh!. I let go of what I knew to be wrong for me, to satisfy his need to feel commitment. At the same time as I did this, the relationship changed. I began to lose respect and deep feelings for him as his truth relating to love and commitment didn't exactly match mine. However, I knew what I was doing and went ahead anyway. Later, we did get engaged, although underneath something had turned me off setting a date for marriage. I couldn't get over the fact that commitment and love for him focused on the material things in life. This was how he felt valued.

In that same year the country was in recession and we were struggling to make ends meet. I was always able to get reasonably high paying jobs, but I also had a yearning to do something with my career. The only way was to move to a different area, where opportunities were more abundant. The job market in Bath wasn't so vibrant, so we planned to move to my home county of Surrey. Luckily with my forces background and mix of skills I was able to get work easily. I had found a good job, one of those 'meant to be' moments of being in the right place at the right time. I was given a three month project to set up a programme of activities for young children. It was a challenge, as I hadn't done anything like this before. I was given a blank sheet and a budget to work with. I thrived on the test and succeeded in creating a programme that was to become the backbone for the survival of the business through the recession. They gave me a permanent contract and I stayed on with the company, getting a promotion soon after.

For Steve it was a little different, he didn't find a job so quickly, so we moved in stages. I moved to start my new three month project first and stayed with my parents. Steve was to stay and sell the house and then move to be with me. It made sense, as he hadn't found a job in the new area yet. He would be on hand to look after the house, continue working and move up when the house had gone. In the meantime, I would come back at the weekends to spend time with him.

The plan sounded great on paper, however when it came down to it, Steve became incredibly possessive and really bereft when I left to work in Surrey during the week. He insisted that he needed my car so he could get around town in Bath. This was ludicrous as he could walk to work, whereas I had a good thirty minute drive. But for some reason, it was more important in his eyes that he had the car. Yet another material need that mattered more than mine. We argued about this, as I was the main bread winner and had a longer travel distance to work and it was winter time, cold and snowy. I let him have the car as I didn't like the aggression that came my way. It was better to shut up and let him have his way. I duly went backwards and forwards by train, having to change twice to get to my destination in the cold of winter. It would take me an hour and half, when it should have taken just a quick thirty minute drive by car. I let it go and yet again it was another sign that turned me off him. I gave up expressing myself and started to shut down. Like my marriage before and in a different way, I didn't like what I had become in this relationship.

As time went on, I wasn't able to let go of Steve's attitude and it played on my mind. Unresolved feelings were just beneath the surface and there was an underlying rift between us. It seemed that the time apart strengthened his possessiveness and strengthened my resentment. I didn't realise at the time that this was heading me into a direction I really needed to go in.

After I got awarded the permanent contract, the house in Bath sold quickly and I began to think that all of our insecurities and niggles were due to the change and upheaval, so we went ahead and moved. We bought a house that needed some love and attention and focussed on building a new life. I was hoping my feelings towards him would rekindle.

I thrived in my job, Steve did okay too and found something he enjoyed doing, but he started to become jealous of my success and as I began to achieve more and more, it drove a further wedge between us. Our sex life diminished and I started to develop all sorts of physical symptoms, knee pain, low back pain, shoulder pain and headaches. I couldn't understand what was wrong with me. The big 30th birthday was looming and I was in pain. I began to resent Steve being around even more and I became very introverted and depressed when I was at home. He was concerned, but I couldn't express myself to him as I didn't know what was wrong. I felt like I couldn't breathe.

Being with Steve gave me the opportunity to start a proper healing, albeit unconsciously. The relationship had given me a sense of stability of sorts so that I felt safe to start to reveal my deeply buried pain.

I decided to go to the doctor. The doctor I saw turned out to be an angel in disguise. He listened to me going on about the pains I had in my body, knees, stomach, shoulders, back pain and calmly said at the end, "So what's the real problem?" It was like a bolt of lightning as if he could see straight through me.

That one question made me squirm inside. I still didn't connect with the problem, but in that moment of discomfort, something unplugged inside and all the old tremors of self-loathing surfaced in a volcano of emotion. Words erupted out of my mouth, words that had not been uttered for years to anyone. "I was raped when I was fifteen!" Uck... that was awful to say.

He was incredible and didn't ask me any details. I think he could see it was very raw and simply said, "Let's get you some help shall we?" Through my tears I shook my head to confirm it was okay. There was such a huge relief inside that I could not put it into words. I walked out of that surgery, red faced, blurry eyed but with a renewed sense of optimism and freedom. Help at last, thank you.

Lightness through the dark

Without thinking, just trusting my gut instinct, I made some immediate changes. I decided to join a swimming club. There was an excellent masters club not far from where we lived. Steve didn't like this one bit, as it was something he couldn't get involved in. My birthday was due and I knew I couldn't bare the torment of being with Steve any longer, for his sake as well as mine. I felt suffocated. No matter how hard it was I had to let go. I couldn't tell him why, as I had no way of articulating what was going on inside for me. I was a mess and couldn't offer him anything. I just had to tell him that my feelings were confused and I no longer wanted to be with him. It was one of the hardest things to do, but I had to do it. He really hadn't done anything wrong, it was all about my own survival. I couldn't offer anyone a truthful relationship without getting to the bottom of my own problem.

I seriously wanted to sort myself out, so that I could enjoy a deep meaningful relationship with a man. I realised I had been living a lie. Shut down and insecure, I couldn't be living any further from the truth. I still wasn't sure what that all meant, but a determined force welled up inside of me to discover that which was missing.

Steve understood that the house we had bought was mainly with my money in the end, but as I was the one wanting to let go of us, I decided it was best that I would leave and go and stay with my parents whilst he found somewhere else to live. I couldn't bear the atmosphere in the house, it made me more miserable and less able to function at work. I made sure I kept my car this time.

Steve took the split very badly, well of course he would. I couldn't give him a valid reason for it and he refused to leave. We had many arguments as he found it hard accept that I didn't want to be with him. It was awful, I really felt for him but there was no turning back for me, I had to get myself sorted out. I knew if I didn't do this I wouldn't be alive for very long. The dark deep wound inside would consume me and lead me down a slippery path, where I could easily go. Whatever I had to do, no one could do for me.

It took nine months of wrangling with Steve. He was quite happy living in the house and having girlfriends around. Eventually and funnily, what did the trick was when I took a loan out and bought him a car. He was as happy as Larry and around the same time he found himself a more serious relationship and left to live with her. I moved back into my house and continued with the restoration on my own, which I found very satisfying.

During this time, my parents were incredibly supportive and my Dad helped me with getting the house restored once Steve had left. I was doing very well at work, that part was at least was normal. My house became my retreat.

It was pure and simple, I was in survival mode. I had really considered not being here on this planet, and even started to fantasise about how to leave. But however wretched I felt about myself, something kept me driving forward. The swimming was therapy, familiar, meditative, fun, hard work and my saviour during this time. The house was a focus to keep me busy at home and work was exhilarating, creative and most of all, I was valued for what I did and the energy that I gave. All these elements kept me going, as underneath I felt I was dying.

I started having four weekly sessions with a specialist rape trauma professional. It was strange, there were lots of silences in the beginning and I sat in session sometimes feeling very awkward, but slowly, very slowly the words came and the feelings came up to the surface. Very gently, he guided me to distinguish between my different feelings, emotions and thoughts. I became an expert on recognising what feelings, emotions and thoughts related to everyday reality and what related to the rape. I began to see a pattern and discern what was normal and what needed conscious attention. Slowly, I got back in touch with the deepest part of me that had buried and disconnected itself all those years ago. No wonder my husband found solace with someone else. I was only functioning on the surface and out of duty.

It was a heavy twelve months of intensive guided self work, but I did well. I reconnected the physical, emotional, mental and spiritual aspect of the part of me that had died on that day. The specialist said he was very pleased with my progress and he felt that I had all the tools to continue healing. I felt absolutely fine. The well of happiness inside of me said it all. Life seemed so much clearer and brighter for a while at least.

It took, four years to get my life into some sort of order. I was single, successful and reasonably happy. I started to dream again of meeting my soul mate. After four years of swimming training, I lost interest after competing in the Masters World Swimming Championships in Sheffield. It was instant, like a light bulb switching off. I came back from the competition with no drive or ambition to swim another length. So I stopped training, thinking the feeling would pass. It had been such a big build up to the championships, but the urge never returned. Later I realised swimming training was therapy in itself, meditation in water if you like. It kept me alive and gave me a form of healing outside of the workplace, which I didn't realise at the time. It left a void, but I had no inkling to fill that void with something else. The next stage of my healing had begun.

After a while, loneliness began to be a big part of my life. I really felt incredibly isolated when I got home at night. There was nothing to fill the empty space with and actually I didn't want to. However, it became too much and to suppress the feeling of emptiness I would buy a bottle of wine, switch on the telly and generally get drunk, fall into bed and sleep it off. This would become a habit.

What was happening? Something was missing. Slowly, the job I loved became less inspiring. It was the same thing every day and every year. The country was going through a severe recession again and my mortgage payments went sky high. I needed to earn good money to keep a roof over my head and I felt trapped again.

Never one to be deterred, I decided to look for another job, something different. I applied for a job as a recruitment consultant which meant regular hours and good money. It was a tough interview process. In fact, the manager at the time later became my best friend and she still is today. I got the job and duly immersed myself into something new. It was a big change. I had complete autonomy in my previous job with a lot of freedom to create potential and manage different personalities. Now, I had to conform to targets and sit at a desk. So, I made the most of getting out of the office to meet potential clients which gave me some sense of freedom at least.

For a while I really enjoyed this new way of working. However, after about six months, the routine became less attractive and the loneliness started to kick in again. I felt like a recluse. I was not a big party goer or socialiser. I loved people and being with people, but was not so interested in going out at night and being surrounded by people I didn't know. I was much happier being with work colleagues.

We had fun in the office, even though the focus was about sales and targets, my friend and manager was great at creating ideas, opportunities and guidance. She herself became disillusioned with the company and eventually left. The job became repetitive and flat and I became disinterested and de-motivated. I only lasted for a year. I missed the creativity and challenge of starting something from scratch and being with like-minded, hardworking people. Recruitment was about suits and targets. There was no 'heart' and without my buddy, it became evident it was not my scene.

Flying away

Feeling lost, I really didn't know what I could do so I took some time out and travelled to Australia, a short trip of about one month. I went with a friend of mine as she had family there. We flew on the mammoth trip to Melbourne, with a short stop in Singapore and a four day trip to Bali. Freedom again, at last.

Bali was incredible, reminiscent of the impact of India, years before but the smell was different. Bali oozed beauty, smiling faces and kindness. It was such a world away from life back home. It was so colourful and the lush green topical plants and trees were rich in colour. Even the dirt was a rich deep red brown. Every thing seemed to have hidden depths. Then there was the humidity. Never in my life had I experienced such stifling 'wet' heat. I quickly acclimatised and actually quite enjoyed the cloying warmth. It didn't bother me that my hair became flat and straight as soon as we went outside and that it was absolutely useless to wear any kind of make up. Everything just melted. My limbs were heavy all the time and it was an effort to walk anywhere far, but it deeply relaxed my body.

As this was a stopover, we only had four days to recover from our journey. The daytime was spent on the beach, where we were pestered by ladies selling their wares. We learned to just ignore them and say no very strongly. They soon realised we weren't big spenders and left us alone to target other unsuspecting tourists who were willing to be pestered constantly. We saw the pattern with other tourists, if you bought one item, it was like bees to honey pot, they never stopped coming.

We went on a trip to a temple high in the mountains. I really don't remember much, just that it was an exceptionally beautiful drive and a far cry from the hustle and bustle of the town and resort areas. It was tangibly serene. The people were beautiful, so soft and kind with lovely smiles. I wondered what was hidden beneath.

Four days later and we boarded the flight to Melbourne. I liked Melbourne and, of course, it was a complete contrast to Bali in every sense. It is a modern cosmopolitan city full of life. I spent a few days with my friends' family then I flew on to Sydney on my own. We were to meet up in Queensland a few days later.

On arrival at the airport in Sydney the most amazing synchronicity occurred. On the flight from London I was sat next to a man in his sixties and his wife. They were just retired and looking forward to their first ever big trip overseas. They were doing the whole thing, a stop off at Singapore then a tour of Australia and New Zealand. They were a lovely couple. About four hours into the trip we were just about to have a meal when he slumped over his food tray. We tried to wake him, but it was obvious something was seriously wrong. He wouldn't come round. I felt for his pulse and checked his breathing. He was still alive. His wife was in shock, bless her. I called the flight attendant who came and had a look, but he wasn't sure what to do so went to ask a colleague. Then an announcement came over the public address system to ask if there was a doctor on board. Luckily there was and he came and checked him over.

My friend and I were moved from our seats, to give more room for the man to lie down. I ended up right at the back of the aircraft. I got the short straw, my friend ended up in business class! It didn't matter to me as I was very worried for the man and his wife. When we stopped off at Singapore, the man had come round and was able to sit up and eventually very slowly was helped off the plane. I prayed that he would be okay. I really felt for both of them.

Anyhow, here I was at Sydney airport waiting for my bags and stood right next door to me was the couple on the plane. He looked amazing. Apparently, he had recovered very quickly in Singapore. No one could tell him what had happened, but he had recovered enough to be given the all clear to continue on his travels. It was such a blessing in disguise as the whole incident had played on my mind and I was now able to let that worry go. We enjoyed a cup of coffee together, said our goodbyes and went our separate ways.

So, here I was in the middle of Sydney, how exciting. The city was alive with vibrancy. Unbeknown to me I had arrived at the start of the gay pride festival of Sydney. I was surrounded by flamboyancy, fun and frolics. I felt incredibly safe and wandered around the city without fear, went to all the famous sites, spent a day on the beach at Manly and generally had a fabulous time. During one of my walking trips, I bumped into another couple that had been on the flight from London. I've always found it amazing that you can be thousands of miles away from home and yet bump into people that you know. It happened earlier in my life on a family holiday to Tangier, we ran into twins who lived a few doors up from us at home. They were staying in the same hotel and we had no idea they were going to the exact same place.

Another four days later and I was on a plane travelling north into Queensland. There I was to meet up with my friend again and we were to spend two weeks based in Port Douglas and enjoy a beach type holiday. Much to our disappointment it rained torrentially for most of that time!

Determined to make the most of it we booked a trip to dive off the Great Barrier Reef. I'd had to take some sea sickness tablets as we were going out on a catamaran. The water was choppy and it was a windy, grey day. About twenty minutes out of the harbour the engines failed. It was my worst nightmare. There was no escape and the motion was too much. The tablets did their trick and I wasn't sick, but I felt terrible and my friend joked with me at my colour, a sort of greyish green. We sat like ducks in the ocean being buffeted by the waves for about forty five minutes whilst waiting for the repair to be done before finally getting underway.

Although the sun didn't shine, it mattered not as I dived down into the ocean. The vision under the water was like a different world. I was in my element. It was so quiet, only the sound of my own breathing. The colours and shapes were incredible. An hour or so earlier I had been in turmoil about taking this trip, particularly when we bobbed up and down stranded on the ocean, but it was well worth the discomfort, the dive was brilliant.

The reason the weather was so bad, was because a cyclone had hit the north coast of Australia and we were getting the remnants of that weather front. It could have been worse. We decided to keep an eye on the weather and duly drove south towards sunshine. There we enjoyed about four days on a sunny beach. It made our two week beach holiday a little more authentic!

On the way home we stopped off at Hong Kong. I was violently ill for the whole two days only managing to see the four walls of my hotel room! My friend did the sight seeing tours for me and she shared her experience with photos.

Travel bug

Arriving back home we were coming into spring time and I seriously wondered what I was going to do with my life. I so loved to travel. The feeling of freedom and frenetic activity at the airports, the unknown, somehow made me feel alive. I really didn't want to get back into a normal routine.

Before going to Australia I had sold my house and bought a smaller one in a more expensive area, but with good opportunities for work. I thought hard about what I knew I excelled at and what made me feel good. The combination of helping people and travel were two key elements. "Mmm, what could I do?"

I decided a good combination was to try and get a job that involved travel and helping people. I got a job as a villa manager in Menorca. It seemed ideal at the time, a short term six month contract, living on a beautiful Mediterranean island in the sun. Menorca was a lovely island, not particularly dramatic in any way, just simple countryside, lovely beaches and crystal clean sea.

The glamour soon turned into reality. It was hard work for six days a week and my day off was spent recovering and washing clothes. I was lucky as I had a car to drive around in, so I did have a lot of autonomy and planned my own day, but the workload was heavy. Meeting and greeting at the airport, visiting clients in villas and sorting out any problems and being on call for emergencies created a very unforgiving environment.

As the season evolved, I found time to go out in the evenings after work. Eating and drinking late was the norm, very similar to Greece. There were four of us sharing the same working region and two of my colleagues had hooked up with some local guys so I felt a bit of a gooseberry going out with them at times. I made the most of the nightlife and met some interesting people, but was happy staying free and single.

Being one of the more mature reps, I was lucky to share a flat with another woman of a similar age. She was a mother to a teenage girl who lived back in the UK. Pam was easy to get on with. In a similar role to me, we were able to share our thoughts and feelings. I came to realise how important it was to have a friend to talk with and share experiences. Existence was very lonely otherwise.

It was a good six month interlude in my life bit I was not sure about making a career of this as by the end of the season I was wacked and ready for a break. I was offered a winter season in Madeira and decided I would do this and then look at pursuing something else. After a week at home, I packed again and flew into Funchal, the capital city of Madeira.

What a difference. Madeira was miles from anywhere, no beaches, an island of mountains, deep ravines and semi tropical climate. Funchal was located in a basin and looked brilliant under the night sky. My base was in a place called Canico, on the outskirts of the city. My role was to visit the more remote outposts, checking in on guests who were staying in hotels far away from the main city area. Depending on the weather the drive to these places was sometimes treacherous. Roads were cut through steep sided walls of solid rock and, when it rained, stones and mud would fall onto the roads. As it was the winter time, this happened frequently.

I managed to see quite a lot of this unique island. I remember driving into a place called the 'Nuns' Valley.' The road ran round the edge of the mountain range, it was high with no protection on one side, taking you through the occasional tunnel of rock. I was scared of heights and had to keep my attention completely focussed on the road. When I did stop at a lay by, the view was breathtaking. The road was so high up the houses of the villages below looked like dots on a map.

The story of the Nuns' Valley is that nuns had settled here many centuries ago whilst they were seeking refuge from frequent pirate attacks. The area is famous for chestnuts and cherries and the famous liqueur, Ginga, made from wild cherries. It must have been an incredible journey for these nuns to make to the valley back in those days as the route would have been treacherous, but necessary for their survival.

In Funchal, where our main office was located, I enjoyed the diversity of being back in a city environment. Having to visit the office everyday, it reminded me of living in London, waiting in rush hour traffic and the smells of city life.

We were coming up to the year end taking us into the new millennium and prepared for the coming of the year 2000. Big celebrations were planned in the city. We planned for emergency contingencies in case everything 'crashed,' as some experts had predicted. I was part of the emergency team that was to stay in the city on New Year's Eve in case we had to rescue guests. Who knew what was going to happen?

In the meantime, it was Christmas. It was a low key affair for us. We shared a lunch with some other company reps and then went back to friends' hotel room to watch a film. Boxing Day was great. We had the day off and got up in the morning, looked out into the brilliant sunshine. It was such a beautiful day for a walk. The quay side was a buzz of energy, coffees shops were open, selling ice cream. Smiling faces were everywhere; yachts were moored on the pontoons with the familiar chinking of sail wires, adding to the magical scene. It was the first time I had experienced Christmas away in the sunshine. So different!

On New Year's Eve we had been invited to a party on the top floor of one of the best hotels in Funchal. The view was spectacular. A number of big cruise liners were peppered around the port, it was going to be a big night. I had to stay sober, of course, as I was on call. The rumours of an amazing firework display were rife, so at midnight waiting for my emergency stand by phone to ring, the fireworks commenced. Funchal became alight with an orchestrated dance of light in the night sky. Fireworks lit up the cruise ships and then systematically, like a symphony, rang out around the basin of the city. At set intervals bursts of energy emerged. It was mesmerising. You felt the explosions deep inside you and no one could speak. It was a truly magnificent show. I've never experienced anything like it since. Thankfully the phone didn't ring and everything passed by with out incident.

The rest of the season tumbled by and I was really looking forward to going home. I'd had enough of the six days a week intensity and needed a rest. I got back to the UK and moved back into my house which I had rented out for a year. I was still trying to find myself and carve out some sort of socially respectable method to earn a living. I did a short term contract selling memberships for a health club that was being refurbished. It was selling a dream, partly off plan. I was glad it was short term. I loved meeting and getting to know people, but I didn't like the pressure of sales – more, more, more. I earned a lot of money during this time but I was glad when it was over.

Now I was at a loss again. What to do with my life? There was still that missing link. The thought of doing what I did before didn't really appeal, although I had the greatest time in the Army and working with the leisure company as a manager. So I got temporary jobs; anything really, administration, executive secretarial and PA positions and spent time travelling mainly in between the Channel Islands and Greek islands. There was such a big gap in my life as I drifted from one thing to another and I couldn't put my finger on it at all. I got bored easily and felt like there was something missing inside of me. I felt disconnected to everyday life. It seemed by going away, doing all these different things, I filled a void.

Eureka!

I saw an advert in a paper. It said, 'Workshop. Discover who you are! Holidays in Greece.' Not one for being open to retreat type things, I didn't know anything about them really, but my perception was of weirdo, airy fairy people getting together dancing and prancing around and not having any boundaries. Anyhow, something clicked inside so I read up on some of the workshops. The people running it all looked pretty respectable and the pictures painted a professional outfit. I took the plunge and decided to go in September. I pre booked a workshop that was all about 'Being Here Now.' Don't ask me why I was attracted to that one but it seemed the most attractive thing to do and didn't involve anything out of my comfort zone.

I was very nervous about going for some reason. I put my two feet forward and off I flew into Athens for an adventure I would be eternally grateful for. I discovered that the people I met were normal people, in society's eyes, professionals, even a magistrate, mums and dads rediscovering who they were, young and mature, all of us there for different reasons. Fortunately, the girl I shared with was great, easy going and grounded and we got on fine.

The centre where we would meet everyday was a short walk through a typical Greek village with white washed houses, bougainvillea draping over walls and bars, vines bursting with grapes and skinny cats scurrying around. It felt so familiar and lovely to greet people in the morning with a "Kalimera, ti kanis?" Old men sat in the square, drinking ouzo giving 'us tourists' hard blank stares. The wonderful deep lines on the women's faces spoke of hidden knowing behind their gaze. There weren't many young Greeks here as they had all gone off to work and live in the lively metropolis of Athens, leaving their parents and grandparents to keep the ancient traditions alive.

I kept myself in the background and just observed slowly integrating with a few people I felt drawn to. One person in particular was a man, possibly in his late sixties. It was hard to tell. Charles had an incredible intensity about him, there was no hiding as his dark, deep eyes could bore straight through you. His hair was white and he had these big bushy white eyebrows and was quite tall with a slim build. He almost looked like a white wizard and reminded me of the doctor I had worked for in Germany. He had similar traits and an unknown depth. Some of the others, mainly the so called, respectable professional types, took a dislike to him. Charles was opinionated about certain subjects and could hold you in a discussion for ages, but there was something about him. An academic, a professor by trade, he was there for his own personal reasons. Because he was different, he became the subject of what I would class as bullying, through gossip and conversation. I didn't like it.

There was a local half marathon run advertised, an annual event to which the retreat centre would supply most of the runners. Between the two centres on the island there were about fifty runners. I decided, after a lot of cajoling, to enter as well. Absolutely foolish! What was I doing? I hadn't run properly for years, surely my body couldn't take it. Well I did it. It was awfully painful, I mean really painful, my legs killed me and I have no idea how I finished. I swore I would never do anything like that again without preparing my body first.

The next day I was in agony. Some of the other runners had received massages, as there were a couple of therapists in the group. Charles sensing that I was in agony, asked if I had received any treatment.

"No I haven't." I answered.

"Would you like me to massage your legs?" he said.

Sensing my hesitation, he said, "I practise something called Lomi Lomi massage. It's an ancient technique that will help to release pain in your body. I will only do the backs of your legs." I thanked him and agreed.

He was true to his word. I could tell Charles had spent some time in preparing the room and the table. There was some lovely Hawaiian music playing, he had dressed himself in a Hawaiian sarong and as he started to massage the backs of my legs using his forearms, I noticed him dancing around the table with a rhythm of movement that matched the strokes. It seemed a bit strange, but my legs felt like they were melting. I began to feel like I was in a different place.

When he finished I thanked him and walked down to the beach. I felt incredibly relaxed. The next four hours I cannot recollect. I fell asleep on the beach and when I got up, the pain in my legs and, in fact, everywhere else had disappeared. It was a truly amazing experience.

The next day at lunch I was sat with Charles. I couldn't believe how that short treatment had made a huge impact on my physical body. Everyone else was still suffering and I didn't have any pain. I asked him about what he had done. He told me a little of how he got into practising Lomi Lomi massage and the ancient philosophy behind the system called Huna. I found this fascinating. My mind was doing overtime. I wanted to know more and I felt very excited for some unknown reason.

He asked me if I worked with energy. I didn't understand him. What did he mean? So he demonstrated. I stood in front of him and closed my eyes and he said to me, "All I want you to do is to focus on how you are feeling."

When I opened my eyes, he said, "What did you sense?"

I said. "I felt anger." Charles had made himself feel angry and I had picked up on the angry energy he was giving off.

Now it clicked. I had become conscious of 'energy' in action. It was a big light bulb moment and connection in my life. I could trust my gut feeling and what I felt was true. I had attended the workshop I had booked onto. That had also left me feeling open and receptive to more than I could understand or comprehend.

The two incidents left me feeling free, alive and clear and wanting to know more. I didn't attend any more of the workshops as I wanted to integrate and revel in this new found reality. Whatever it was, it felt good. Was this the missing link?

I left there after two weeks, returned back to the UK not looking forward to starting a new job. When I got home, I realised the new job really wasn't a good move for me, so I phoned and turned down the position. Now what do I do? I really felt like I wanted to study. Something had happened on that holiday and I needed to change my life around.

That's exactly what I did. I enrolled on a course at a college to learn anatomy and physiology and massage. I had no idea how I was going to fund the course. I just trusted it was the right thing to do. I managed to get a grant to help with the fees, but I still had the problem of supporting myself with a mortgage to pay. I rented out my house and did temporary jobs and moved in as a lodger with a friend of mine. It helped us both out. She needed help to pay her mortgage and I needed to cut down on my outgoings. We shared a house near to the South coast and I loved being near to the ocean.

The next few years were dedicated to studying and personal development. I was hungry for knowledge and hungry to connect to a deeper side of me. I studied an energy based system called Polarity Therapy which covered everything from energy anatomy, bodywork, nutrition, yoga exercises and counselling to emotional processing skills. I then set up a private practise and for the next three years I ran a regular therapy business and met some wonderful people who were going through their own challenges in life and I was privileged to be a part of that journey.

During this time, and after I had completed my Polarity training, I had an urge to visit Hawaii. This was prompted, in part, by my experience with Charles a few years earlier, but also by my teachers in Polarity, who had introduced a method into our training to do with Huna, meaning Hidden knowledge. It was such a strong calling I couldn't ignore it, so much so that I saw a tiny advert in a magazine about a Huna retreat on the island of Maui. It was due to start in three weeks. My heart leapt out of my chest and a strong voice inside of me kept saying that I must go! Based on my previous experience of trusting my gut feeling, I couldn't deny those signs, could I!? I only just had enough money and booked a place on the course and a flight and searched the net for accommodation to cover the two nights before the retreat started. I was going to Hawaii. Was I mad?

RIPPLING WAVES

"A true gift is one which has taken time to create with love in your heart and a story to tell with or in its creation"
Hawaiian Man on a Maui beach

On the edge

The wind was howling in my Victorian flat. It was a cold dark and stormy winter night. I went outside to deposit the trash and place the bin on the pavement ready for collection the next morning. As I came back into the house a sharp gust of wind slammed shut one of the inside doors with a bang. The glass shattered and I felt something warm at the back of my left leg. I pulled up my trouser leg and a shard of glass was sticking out from top of my left calf. I didn't feel any pain, just warmth from the blood now flowing out of the wound. I promptly removed the glass shard, which I probably shouldn't have, and wrapped my leg in a tea towel. After examining the wound, it wouldn't stop bleeding. I started to worry about how deep it could be, all I could think about was what if it had caused some underlying damage that would prevent me from flying. A surreal thought really. It was seven days away from a trip of a lifetime to Hawaii.

I took myself off to the nearest hospital to get it checked out. Thankfully it wasn't as bad it looked, I had a couple of stitches and was sent on my way. It healed quickly and by the time I left, the hole in the back of my leg had sealed and there was a small half inch new red scar over the wound. The ferocity and directness of that impact, made me wonder what it was all about. It was almost as if someone was trying to tell me something! I had learned that good and bad things happen for a reason.

I had been living on the isle of Portland for six months, after moving out of the house that I shared with my friend so as to reclaim some space of my own. I rented a ground floor flat with a sea view overlooking Chesil Beach in Dorset. It was fantastic. The weather was extreme. I loved watching the weather fronts roll in over the ocean and embrace the beautiful evening sunsets. It was a most dramatic setting.

My everyday ritual was to take an early walk down to the pebbled beach, sit, watch, listen and then quiet my mind to meditate by the ocean. There I would be joined by a playful sea lion, which had one day appeared, emerging from the seaweed a few metres off the beach area by the rocks. We stared at each other for a long while. His eyes were glistening, dark and enormously kind looking. Then he would proceed to show me how clever he was in the water, diving in and out over the waves, disappearing for what seemed like age, only to re-emerge in another place and then turning to see if I was looking. He was very cheeky. He felt like a 'he' and not a 'she,' although I wouldn't have known the difference and it didn't matter. I'm sure he thought I was a little strange as I practised some breathing and yoga stretching exercises and made silly sounds as I did so. We were buddies for a while, until one day he didn't turn up anymore. It was a wonderful interaction. It made me remember the close connection we all have with animals and took me back to my younger days and the close bond I had with mine.

My business was building well and although Portland was further away from my place of work, it didn't matter that I had longer journey. The very nature of my work as a practitioner was absorbing and I needed space to be in an environment close to nature, which enabled me to clear and rejuvenate myself, ready to feel refreshed for the next day.

To the back of my home were the steepest cliffs and hills. There were a couple of walks I would take. One was up a green grass slope going directly north east towards the old battlement bunkers, left over from the war, and the other up was around a rocky pathway to the cliffs facing south. Both areas held very different and particular energies and sensations. From the cliff walk I would feel exhilarated and refreshed but from the battlement walk a heaviness and deep sense of foreboding. On a warm sunny day the battlement walk would feel fine, but on other days it would feel inhospitable and I would just want to run through the area very quickly. Needless to say, I didn't do that walk very often and only when the sun was shining. Sensing the difference in the places helped me to tune in to what was around me and the environment even more. I realised the power of the elements and the way they can change a mood or feeling. Even the densest of forms such as rocks and stones held a kind of essence, that could be related to something almost tangible in a feeling sense. I recognised that the environment I chose to live in was extremely important for my overall well being.

Portland was a sort of training ground, preparing me for my next adventure. In a much more vivid and profound way, living there taught me respect for the power of nature and the land. The sense that anything could happen at any moment which could change a current reality, like the shard of glass incident, created from just a strong gust of wind. By taking the time to open up and sense what was around I, yet again, learned not to be afraid as choices were always available. Life was good, solitary but good. I earned a living doing what I loved to do, lived in a place that supported me physically and energetically and now I was ready to experience more. The islands of Hawaii beckoned.

A new era

I was so excited when I left London, so unbelievably grateful for this opportunity. I was only going for ten days. It was half way round the world, such a long way, but I didn't care. It felt absolutely right.

I arrived in Hawaii on the same day I left London, twenty hours plus of travel time, eleven hours behind Greenwich Mean Time. The best part of the journey was getting on the plane at San Francisco for the five hour flight to Kahului in Maui. The sun was setting and as we flew away from the continent. I looked below in awe at the rippling waves of the ocean way below and a few dotted puffy cotton ball clouds in the sky. The enormity of this journey hit me. It was such an expanse of water, so remote and so blue. As we left the land the clouds became few and far between, the sun slowly disappeared and the night sky emerged showcasing brilliant dazzling stars that lit up the universe. We flew for five hours over the Pacific. Finally, I arrived in one of the most remote groups of islands on the planet. Something deep inside began to really stir. What I had felt I was missing for so long, in an intangible sense, was beginning to re-establish a link.

It was around eight in the evening, dark and balmy warm. My first memories were of a fragrant smell in the air and the sounds of zebra doves cooing their song. Tired and jet lagged I found my way to the rental car compound, collected my car and navigated my way in an automatic left hand drive across to the other side of the island. A tricky scenario. I was tired, it was my first time in a new place and I had never driven an American automatic left hand drive before. It was pitch black and I had about an hour to drive to my accommodation. I had been lucky to get anywhere to sleep as when I booked back in the UK, accommodation availability was tight and there was very little choice. Lahaina, the commercial town of the island, became my first port of call. I eventually found the hotel after an anxious drive and I slumped into a deep sleep.

Waking early in the morning, bleary eyed and suffering the effects of a long journey, my excitement took over. I got myself together and walked outside to see Maui for the first time. It was a lovely warm soft early morning. I took a stroll down to Front Street in Lahaina, and on the ocean side I found a beautiful spot which overlooked the sea of glistening silvery light and had breakfast. I tasted the delights of fresh tropical fruit and good clean wholesome food. People were smiling, Aloha! Everyone was so friendly and open. I felt immediately at home and fully connected. This was paradise, bright colours, rolling waves and a sense of homecoming filled me with happiness. After breakfast I took a walk along the street and came across this enormous, and I do mean enormous, Banyan tree. I thought to myself, "Isn't nature amazing." This old tree was a canopy for those in need of shelter from the intensity of the sun. The tree canopy and roots played host to an array of creative individuals, who were showcasing their work and hoping to sell to admiring passers by.

I sat with the tree for an hour or so, watching people coming and going and very slowly, not conscious of time anymore I made my way to the beach area. I knew a swim in the ocean and a lie on the beach would help my body get into form following such a long flight. I found a palm tree to relax under and a beautiful lagoon to wallow in. I really was in paradise.

I stayed there most of the day. Laying on the earth is one of the only things that truly helps me 'ground'. It was late afternoon and I was thinking about getting back to my hotel, when I noticed this handsome Hawaiian man with his beautiful young daughter, picking things out of the sand and placing them into a bucket. They came near and struck up a conversation. I asked him what he was collecting and he said,

"I am collecting tiny shells to make a necklace for my wife. A true gift is one which has taken time to create with love in your heart and a story to tell with or in its creation."

"What a beautiful thing to say," I thought.

Out of the blue and without any prompting, he said "You should spend a couple of years here. There is plenty of work."

After he left my eyes filled up with tears and my heart felt like it would burst as I imagined being here all the time. I longed for someone to share it with. I will never forget that moment. It was inspiring, and somehow this man's' words touched so many cords inside of me, particularly the part about creating something with love in your heart. It is such a profound truth as when you do create a life with love in your heart, everything does flow.

I began to remember the difference between when I had done things out of a sense of duty or social conditioning, and when I had done things because it felt good. Like the trip to Greece, which was being in an environment that nourished my soul, everything flowed and the fear disappeared. Doing a job that I loved to do, like teaching and practitioner work, which fulfilled my purpose in helping people, rather than a job that didn't inspire or make my heart sing, was so much better than sitting in a stuffy office. Being in a rigid structured routine wasn't for me. A stirring moment, as I realised there are no limits when you follow what feels good deep inside and anything really is possible, even when all you can see are blocks. I began to become conscious of all the times that I had followed my heart but at the same time thinking, I shouldn't be doing this, because of leaving family, friends, or job. However, when I looked back, my action of following my gut feeling lead me to be a much better person and actually, equally as important, benefited those around me too. The world is as large or as small as your own perception.

I went back to the hotel as I was feeling very tired and relaxed around the pool before having a shower and going out for something to eat before bed. The next day I checked out of the hotel and went in search of the retreat centre, where I was to spend the rest of the week. The centre was on the North shore. This area was different in many ways, less commercialised, greener and slightly cooler. It was located on the wetter side of the island. After a long search I finally found the turning off down a track to the place I was to share with another group of people whom I had never met before.

The centre was set in beautiful tropical gardens, mainly uncultivated, and the plants just held back by the wooden frame structured buildings that would house our rooms and workshop area. It was in a truly magnificent location at the top of a ravine with a stunning view of the ocean. In a lawned area, there was hammock strung between two trees and a hot tub, which you could relax in and watch the whales in the distance, or the stars at night. There was also a crystal clear pool to cool off in when the midday sun got too much. Down in the ravine were flowing waterfalls and pools.

Baptism of fire

The group started to arrive and we gathered by the pond, under a pergola and there I met my fellow companions for the week. A real mix of people and all had travelled far from the UK. We were introduced to each other and then shown around the grounds and facilities. Thankfully it was a small group of just eight.

The accommodation was fantastic. I shared a room with another woman, an interesting lady, an osteopath by profession; we had quite a lot in common. Luckily we were upstairs and my bed was directly beneath a glass skylight window. At night it was like sleeping outside as all I could see was the night sky dotted with millions of stars, lending itself to a feeling of limitless possibility. I would lie for hours at bedtime, just getting lost in the universe.

I was drawn to a man in the group. His name was Basho and we seemed to be on a similar wavelength. We enjoyed each others' company. He was a sensitive man, fun, talented, intelligent and respectful. He told me he was gay. We became really close and Basho is still today one of my best friends, even though we live in different locations and don't see each other much, we still sense and share a deep connection from our meeting.

The workshop was intense on many different levels. I felt like I was being opened up to so many possibilities and realities, all very familiar in a way that I could not describe. My senses heightened and I felt good. On the very first day of the workshop, in the evening, we did something called a *'Higher Self' healing meditation. Our facilitator chanted and at one particular part, what I can only describe it as a sudden shot of energy burst into my body through the right side of my chest. It jolted me and immediately I started to cry and it seemed like I wouldn't stop. I couldn't put any emotion to it, it wasn't painful but felt like I had been opened up or injected with something incredibly fine, I couldn't find words for it. Suddenly the crying stopped and I felt great. Every day I was there I experienced some sort of profound awakening, some of which I am unable to find the words to describe. It was reminiscent of the incident a week or so before with the piece of glass in the back of my leg, such a shock of intensity, yet no pain.

Each of us experienced different aspects of ourselves. Sometimes it was annoying as others went through the games and processes that would become a focus of everyone's attention. Of course, we are all entitled to express ourselves in different ways but I found it a challenge when you have so much going on inside yourself and yet you have to hold it all together for the good of the group. That is what it was like for me, rightly or wrongly. However, I realised much later on, that it was a blessing in disguise to share this experience. It simply wouldn't have been the same on my own. Whatever was going on for one, you could be sure it was resonating at some level with all of us. That's why at the time it felt frustrating, as so much more was going on at much subtler levels for all of us. The power of a group energy is immense.

We shared some wonderful light and beautiful moments. One day half of our group went out on a small rubber motor boat. Yes, another boat ride, urgh. Please keep me free from feeling sick I thought. We went out with a local guy called Randy, who was a whale conservationist. Randy didn't agree with the big commercial boats taking people out to the whales and chasing them so the tourists could take photos, which actually was against the law. He much preferred the laid back approach, so we spent the morning snorkelling. The longer I was in the water the better, being on the boat bobbin up and down in the ocean swell would set the uneasy sickness feelings off.

Finally, we set off for the open water. I sat right at the front of the boat, so I could see the horizon and get blasted by the wind flowing through my hair. It was exhilarating. We slowed and stopped for a bit and in the distance there was a whale and her cub swimming away from us. We waited. Basho started to sing. He had a beautiful voice and incredibly the whale and her cub turned and came towards us. She came close then dived under our boat. It was a truly incredible experience. We were speechless and in awe of her grace, beauty and trust. It had made our day. My feelings of sea sickness completely disappeared. It was an absolute privilege to have been so close to such an ancient animal of the sea who had trusted and graced us with her presence. A reminder yet again of when our hearts are open we become more aware of the deepest connection we have with other beings on this planet. When we do things unconsciously it results in the greatest of harm we can manifest for all. This was truly an emotional and very heart warming moment and a reminder that we have a huge responsibility to look after our planet, lest we destroy the beauty and therefore our fellow friends.

Pushing boundaries

One Sunday late afternoon near to the end of our week, we drove to a huge beach and trekked along to the end, climbed up a cliff and over the hill to a secret bay beach area. Not all of our group were completely able bodied but we somehow managed to get everyone over and emerge onto this colourful beach scene.

The beach was full of people, some were naked, some were dressed as hippies. There were all manner of frivolities taking place, yogis doing yoga, jugglers juggling, musicians playing, a fire burning and a sense of free love in the air. Then there were the drums. A sense of excitement and incredible energy building up from a tribal rhythm that seemed to reverberate deep inside every cell of your body. As a group we must have looked quite odd converging onto this celebration. A couple of the more mature ladies in our group had umbrellas to shade them from the sun and some weren't dressed for the beach at all. It was a little Victorian scene of English eccentricity.

Anyhow, Basho and I looked at each other and without a word, immediately took the opportunity to make the most of the sunshine and sea and stripped off down to our costumes and ran laughing into the huge surf of the Pacific Ocean. The waves were immense. In amongst our frivolity a deep sense of knowing swept over me. This could be potentially dangerous so I kept my consciousness fully alert for the ever changing movement and tide of the ocean, as it felt extremely powerful. I knew that you should never turn your back on the ocean.

At one point, bobbing up and down in the depth of the ocean we stopped and looked back at the beach. We laughed so much it hurt, in the nicest possible way. The vision was truly amazing. Our group stuck out like a sore thumb, the quintessential English image of quiet reserve, wonderfully accepted by those around. Differences didn't matter here.

This gathering was a weekly ritual, open to all, whether you were a Kama'aina, a native of Hawaii or someone who had lived there a long time, or just a visiting tourist. Not for the faint hearted, but an opportunity for people to share and be free from social constraints and judgements. You could be who you wanted to be, knowing at all times it was your choice. People danced around the camp fire as the sun started its slow descent. In honour of the sun's warmth and light that it brings everyday, a hula dancer was stood on a rock away from the beach and silhouetted against the fading light, she carried out a mesmerising dance. Her movements were intoxicating, soft and flowing, like a magician bringing in the magic of the night sky.

The next day we took a trip to a place called 'Iao Valley, a sacred valley and you could feel it. Here I was to have another amazing experience. Driving through a ravine, going deep in towards the valley, there was a feeling of ancient knowledge engrained in every stone and rock. It was as if the majestic, steep mountains either side were speaking. It took your breath away as everything became deep and quiet, bar the sounds of nature.

'Iao Valley is the site of one of the Hawaii's most famous battles, the battle of Kepaniwai, the damming of the waters, in 1790 when King Kamehameha I destroyed the Maui army of Kalanikupule, his son, in an effort to unite the Hawaiian Islands. This was one of the first confrontations in the islands with the use of cannon. It is said that the 'Iao stream ran red with blood all the way to the ocean and that the number of warriors fallen held back the waters of the river, thus the name given to the battle.

With nothing but the deepest respect in our hearts, we walked down along the whispering stream and in amongst the guava trees and other tropical plants. Being conscious of each step, the potential for anything to happen here was evident in everything. Stopping in an area where we could easily bathe in the cool stream water, we continued with our lessons and learned about resonating with the elements. After our session, we spent some time sharing a packed lunch, enjoying the sunshine streaming through the trees.

I sat quietly on the boulders a little apart from the others and watched the ever flowing stream rumble down from the heights of the mountains above. I was looking across to the other side of the stream when I saw something that made me tingle with excitement, and this is going to sound crazy, and I am not crazy although after seeing this I thought I could be, it looked like an elf or something, about three foot tall with big ears and hairy. He had turned round to look at me with a smile on his face, before springing off through the deep foliage. I took in a sharp breath and turned around to see if anyone else had noticed, but it seemed like I was in a different reality all together. My vision was weird and misty and I had to snap myself back and focus on the people in our group. I tried to say with excitement, "Did you see, did you see." But no words would come out, so I kept it to myself.

Later that evening when I reflected on the day, it reminded me of that time in the Army on exercise when I thought I saw things moving in the night, maybe I really had seen something then! Anyway, that would not be the last time I would have similar experiences in this sacred place. The veil here was very thin, lending a way to see the unthinkable. I began to recognise that my sensitivities, as a child, were really a blessing. I was able to perceive and be open to different realities that were beyond our everyday belief systems and limits. I felt so grateful in that moment for my parents and all of my good and bad experiences. They had enabled me to get to this point in time, where the puzzle of Life began to chink into place. I no longer needed to fearful or be anxious, as in the process of letting go of what is known, new energies and life flows in.

I was no longer disconnected, wondering what I was missing in life. My trip here, driven by a deep desire, had re-established that long lost link at the most profound level. I recognised that my perceptions and visions were real. It was a blessing, to be able to sense and see that which is hidden on many different levels. This was yet another doorway opening into many new experiences to come and a reminder that we live in a duality of life in every sense. If we choose we can be enriched by both the physical and metaphysical planes of existence.

The week ended all too soon and it was time to prepare for the long journey back to the UK. I spent the last day with my new found friends from the course and we enjoyed a day of beach, shopping and eating at our favourite restaurant. I really didn't want to go back. Island living suited me.

The flight was long and uneventful. Arriving back, however, I found my suitcase had been broken into and all the mementos as gifts I had purchased from Hawaii were gone. In amongst my devastation, a mischievous thought came into my mind. "That's it I've got to go back, if only to bring gifts back for my family and friends!"

Outside it was cold, busy and hectic. Back with a bump, I found it really hard to adjust. The suitcase incident was the icing on the cake as far as my discontent was concerned as I thought of the people who had done it, coupled with the fact that I didn't know who I was anymore. I had just experienced such an alternative way of being, how on earth could I manage to integrate this into my daily reality back here? I was so thankful to be living near the sea in the UK, it drew me and as the days passed, I made time to watch the sea, dreaming of Hawaii, not knowing if I would ever be able to venture back there again.

Connection

It took me a good few weeks to fully reintegrate as the trip had such a profound effect on me and I had never experienced jet lag like it. The good thing was that my practise thrived when I returned and I was able to offer much more than I had before, in terms of energy understanding and healing. Even more so, after meeting that wonderful Hawaiian man on my first day, it made me dream of meeting my soul mate and share my life with someone who sang and created from their heart too. Was there such a person?

I'd been back a couple of months and it was nearing the end of our summer when I met a guy in a coffee shop. It wasn't the coffee shop that I normally frequented, but as I sat down, we caught each others eyes, so I smiled and we just started chatting. He seemed interesting and we had both shared common ground, both having been in the Army. That familiar camaraderie, humour and connection was there plus some kind of electricity happening between us. We agreed to meet up for coffee the following week. I began to get excited and couldn't wait to see him again.

The next time we met, he told me he was married, although he wasn't very happy. "I've heard that one before!" I thought. This was the first guy I had met for a very long time where the sparks flew just sitting next to each other. It had been a long time since I met someone and this one wasn't available. I was deeply disappointed, there was to be no future, what a shame. Knowing there was nothing in this for me on a deeper level, I enjoyed his company and we continued to share a coffee and a chat now and then and stayed in contact, sporadically, for a few months.

Then we lost contact. A few years later, out of the blue he made contact. He was going through his divorce. Talk about timing. I had just met someone and I was living in a different country so I wasn't available! I look back sometimes and think that he could have been the one, but the timing was all out. There must have been some kind of karmic process going on with us!

All I really wanted was to give and receive love from someone special in my life, someone who could commit, someone who would cherish me, not for what I had or for what I did, a person to share my life with. My relationships so far hadn't been that successful, but they had taught me a lot about my own patterns and enabled me to see myself in a much clearer way about my role within these interactions and the choices I had made. They prompted me to work on myself, to give a potential love a chance by processing and releasing the bad experiences from the past.

January came, things were going really well with my business and I had reached my limit with the number of clients I wanted and felt happy seeing. I didn't want to burn myself out and become just another robot practitioner. However, deep inside, an uncontrollable yearning began to emerge to return to Hawaii. I never thought I would be able to get back there. As my business grew I realised that I needed to do some more work on myself in order to be a better practitioner for my clients. I had no idea at this time how I could manage to do that. I had already done an enormous amount of study and personal development over the years. I had a lot to process! But I just knew that I needed another good clear out. The pull to go back to Hawaii became stronger and stronger as the New Year emerged. How could I get there again?

As these thoughts were processing through my mind, I came across an article about Lomi Lomi massage and then I remembered my experience in Greece during the retreat. That was it! I could learn a new skill in Lomi Lomi massage and go to Hawaii to train! The pull got stronger, it was almost painful. I didn't have a lot of money as I lived week by week.

I searched on the internet for a Lomi Lomi training course and right away one presented itself in Maui. It was happening in June, six months away. My mind went into overdrive as it felt absolutely right to go again. How could I earn enough money to go, I thought? I decided to take an additional job. The extra cash made the dream come alive. Knowing that I would have the money to go I went ahead and booked on the course.

I can't really remember too much about the month leading up to me leaving, it went so quickly and before long I found myself on a flight again to Hawaii. The trip was very familiar this time. I knew exactly where to go and what to do. I had booked out fifteen days as I couldn't afford to be away from my practise much longer than that .

Whirlwind romance

Having learned from my trip last time, I allowed three days, before the course started, to get used to the climate and energy of the island again. I found a bed and breakfast to stay in, on the outskirts of Lahaina. It was one of the only ones with availability in my price range. I immediately felt at home and relished the thought of free time to explore all the wonderful places I had visited last time.

The three days went quickly and all the time I kept thinking, "I wish I could share this experience with someone." My heart opened easily here, the beauty, fragrant smells and happy people made it a pleasure. On the third day I checked out of my B & B and decided to go to the beach for the day before finding my way to the retreat centre ready to start the mammoth ten day intensive Lomi Lomi course.

It was a stunningly beautiful day. The surf was up and the ever changing powerful waves were great to play in. The beach was fairly vibrant with energy, but I still had a good space of my own. As I ate my lunch of a tropical fruit salad, I noticed this gorgeous looking guy, sat in a beach chair, looking like a king. He was fit; around six foot tall, tanned and obviously not a tourist. Anyhow, I thought it would be nice to have company and the next minute, as though he read my mind, he got up and walked over and said, "Would you like to share some of my lunch?" It had just been a thought! I couldn't believe it as this blue eyed man strolled over and sat next to me on the sand.

We spent the next couple of hours relaxing, chatting and swimming in the sea. The feeling between us was very strong. Adam's energy seemed to resonate with every pore in my body, a bit like the guy in the coffee shop. His eyes were intense. He had perfect skin and teeth and obviously he spent a lot of time on himself. Instead of thinking, "Is he good enough for me?" an old pattern of doubts crossed my mind as I thought, "Why would a drop dead gorgeous looking man be interested in me?" He was single, having been divorced about two years and had a young child. He had his own business and owned a couple of houses that he rented out. He told me that he had previously been a child star actor and although enjoying what he did now, wanted to get back into films and television. I could certainly see him on a film set. I fleetingly thought he was a little self obsessed with his looks and this was all too good to be true and there must be something wrong? Warning bells were jangling inside, but I wasn't listening to them. My heart was singing and my boundaries were grey. It had been a long time since I met anyone and I was excited. My heart opened and any common sense went out of the window!

It was getting time for me to leave, and it was incredibly difficult to say goodbye to this man. He was engaging. He asked me to come and stay with him and not go to the retreat. I felt torn in two. I mean, I had only just met the guy and he was asking me to give up a course that I had travelled half way round the world to do. Didn't he get that? Hadn't he been listening to me? He didn't want me to go. The conflict raged inside of me, but I had an obligation to myself to do this workshop and was determined to go. Phew, thank goodness I stood my ground. I somehow knew if I had gone with him, I would have been desperately disappointed with myself. So we parted. He took down the details of where I was staying and I had his number, we were to keep in touch somehow. I thought that would be the last I saw of him.

I arrived at the retreat centre, a different one to last time, bigger but just as beautiful with wonderful gardens to wander around. I had a single room, out of the way from the main house, but private and lovely. The group was big. I was the only person outside of the United States to attend and I felt slightly out of place. These people were so confident and open and I seemed like a mouse compared to them.

I soon adapted and mingled and slowly got to know who was who and connected with two people in particular, one was a guy called Gerry. The Lomi Lomi course was incredible. I absolutely adored this modality of working with people. The sacredness of the rituals surrounding the sessions was powerful and loving. My Polarity training and massage practise had put me in a good space for this and it seemed the most natural thing in the world for me to be doing.

The next evening I received a call from Adam. I thought I would never hear from him again, so I was surprised. He couldn't wait to see me. When was I free? Being open and not thinking, I told him I would be free most evenings. This opened a door for a love affair to flourish in the short window of time that I had. He lived on the other side of the island so it was a good hour to get to me and he would come and pick me up in the evening and we would go for something to eat. Later on during the first week, he stayed over in my room. I wasn't entirely comfortable about this arrangement, although I had a single private room I still felt uneasy bringing someone outside of the group into the centre. It reminded me of the many times, I hadn't felt sure about something yet went ahead anyway, only to realise that I should have listened to my indecision which was a protective mechanism for me. I never said anything though. For me, this was too good to be true and I didn't want to spoil the magic. It was a head over heart thing. He would leave in the morning when we were doing yoga. I couldn't understand why no one saw him. He didn't hide and he wasn't exactly a shrinking violet and would certainly stand out in a crowd, but no one saw him.

Adam, started to express his feelings. He couldn't be away from me. He loved me. Could I extend my stay? It was happening so quickly, I felt bombarded and couldn't quite articulate the mixture of feelings and emotions running through me, so I stayed calm and allowed it to unfold, not sure of any boundaries anymore. Underneath, my mind was working overtime. Was this real? So many questions and so much intensity, doubts crept in.

Our time together was really about him. I never really spoke much about what I wanted in life. I couldn't quite see that at the time, it was all so lovely or so I thought. Instead of stopping and saying to him I wasn't sure about any of this, as it was too soon, too fast, and I wanted to focus on the course, I didn't say anything. The pull of the islands was so great that I would have given up anything to stay.

In complete contrast, and talking about synchronicity and the choices available, there was Gerry. We got on well and he would definitely have been someone I would have enjoyed getting to know better but the opportunity or space for that to happen was not available. From the little I knew about him, he could well have been a better partner for me. There was a connection between us the moment we met, but I was so besotted with Adam that I pushed that away. I was looking through rose tinted glasses. Gerry and I didn't get to work with each other during the course, something kept us apart. Perhaps that would have changed everything, but the opportunity didn't arise. Amazingly, he was to pop back into my life a few years later on.

This whole scenario seemed a little like déjà vu. It was very reminiscent of when I got married. There were two men around then, both very different, yet I chose the risky one then and got bitten. Was I about to repeat the same pattern? All my dreams of a romance, a magical feeling of wanting to share this incredible experience were coming true. I was falling for Adam. Was he really serious though? Had I not learned a thing!? I somehow knew what I was doing and I chose not to act on my inners instincts again. I just wanted the fairytale. That inner core strength in valuing my worth, of which I was consciously aware, was there but the conviction of expression wasn't quite strong enough yet.

The day before I left to go back to the UK Adam wanted to know if I was ever going to come back. How could I stay away? This felt like home to me, but I didn't know when or how. He then dropped a bombshell and told me if I came back, I could stay with him and he would help me find work. I said, "Are you serious?" He was deadly serious and we made some plans. I left there on cloud nine, thinking that my boat had come in and that all my dreams were coming true. I still hadn't expressed my needs in any real depth to him. In fact, I actually wasn't sure what they were, but that didn't matter. I thought things would sort themselves out. I was sure of it. I would be back within three months, with that message from the Hawaiian man on the beach, about staying here for a couple of years, ringing in my years.

So it was that the deception of Maui's dream was destined to fulfil its promise in the rippling waves of love.

Higher Self – In ancient Hawaiian wisdom, the Higher self is the super conscious mind/soul and our truth.

BREAKING WATER

"You are not only responsible for what you say, but also for what you do not say"
Martin Luther

Heartfelt extremes

I was on a complete high when I got back and couldn't stop thinking about a new life in Hawaii. I also couldn't believe my luck. I had fallen in love with a gorgeous looking guy who lived in Hawaii, the place of my dreams and where I felt most at home. The connection I held with this ancient land, was so strong, my soul was singing. It seemed not to matter how I would get to be there.

It was summer time and we were experiencing fabulous weather in the UK. The white sandy beaches of the south coast could almost make you believe you were in paradise. I didn't see or really embrace the beauty around me, as my heart and mind were in a turmoil as the practicalities of my choice crowded in. Was this really happening? Every fibre in my body was screaming at me to go. My mind was fretting about the logistics of my life here, leaving my family, friends and business. How would that feel? How could I leave everyone and all my worldly goods? My mind was a constant merry go round of confusion. Yet, deep below the surface was an unfathomable drive for me to let go of my life here. There was not an ounce of fear in the decision once I had made up my mind. There was grief and guilt for leaving, but not fear.

I had made up my mind and now I was in overdrive to make it happen. Adam continued to call me from Hawaii on a regular basis, as I made plans to sell up and let go of everything I had to follow a dream to paradise. I hadn't really thought much about how I was going to get a visa as Adam had assured me it would be no problem. In fact, everything seemed not to be a problem. Memories flooded back to me about the time I went the Greece unprepared. But I put it out of my mind, as this time was different, I told myself, I wasn't alone.

The next couple of months, I focussed on selling everything I owned. My best friend helped me and we had a great time filling up my car and taking it to the car boot sales and having fun bartering with people. Some stuff was quite hard to see go, particularly my very oldest Thelwell pony books that I was given as a child. That was a wrench. It was like I was on a mission, those around me thought I was mad. "How can you let everything go?" "How can you leave your family? What about your car? What about your practise? What about your house?" They were right in some way. Saying goodbye to my clients was awfully difficult. I had made plans to refer them on to another trusted therapist, but it's like saying goodbye to your children and letting them go.

In our family, it was a huge time of change. At the same time my sister was also making plans to live a different alternative life with her husband in Ireland. They had bought a cottage that needed a lot of restoration work, but it had the land they wanted for her animals. Her dream was coming true also. The difference was, that they had been planning this for a year and preparations were made to move their home to another place, whereas I was letting go of everything and leaving with a suitcase to a virtually unknown entity!

As we were leaving about the same time, I arranged for a family get together at Mum and Dads. My sister and brother hadn't spoken in years and it was quite something that we were altogether on a sunny Sunday at the end of August. Mother had recently had her knees operated on and was recovering, so she hobbled around on crutches. It was sad to see her in so much pain and that was pulling on me. However, it was a beautiful summer day. We shared a lunch and got out all the old photos of our childhood days. It turned out to be a very pleasant nostalgic time indeed. As it turned out, Mums knee operations were for the very best all round, so I was grateful that seeing her in pain didn't stop me.

I knew everyone thought I was crazy, but they were used to me going off doing out of the norm things. How could I turn down this opportunity? My heart was set and nothing was going to change my mind now! It wasn't as if I didn't have a place to go, or potential opportunities and I was going to be with someone that I thought I loved, what more could I want! My self-deception was working well.

Illusion and warning bells

A week before I was due to leave the UK, I was with my friend Basho in London. We were sharing some time together before I left when I received a call on my mobile from Adam. He sounded different.

"What's wrong?" I asked.

"I don't know how to tell you this," he said, "but I have met someone else."

I went cold. "What do you mean you've met someone else?"

He went on to tell me about her, saying he wasn't sure if it was serious, but he wanted to explore the possibility.

Then he said, "Are you still coming?"

I said, "Well yes, I've sold everything to come over and my flight is booked."

It was like being hit in the stomach with a sledgehammer. Panic rose in side. What was I going to do? I was gob smacked. Had he been lying to me all this time? Why did he keep calling and telling me everything was going to be great? It didn't make sense. It was a complete contrast from what I had been hearing from him.

Yet another deja vu situation, reminiscent of how I felt when I was in the car with my Dad on my way to getting married. I had the same feeling of not being sure of what to do. My heart sank. Again, just the same as before, I didn't even think of backing out. My flights were booked, I had let go of everything and I didn't even own a car anymore. I couldn't back out now. I felt empty at the thought of staying put here in the UK.

I wasn't really listening to anything he said after that. I was incensed and sad, so I put the phone down. On the one hand, I realised in my wanting something so badly, I had put all my eggs in one basket to follow my heart and my dream. You could say I had not looked after myself at all in preparing the groundwork, both with the relationship and the practicalities. This would also seem to be so ludicrous, the enormity of change that I had created in my life had transpired from what was essentially a holiday romance and being blinded by an untruthful relationship. Simply put, I had not placed any boundaries for my integrity to be honoured. Had I allowed myself to be deceived and more importantly had I deceived myself, or was there something else at play? On the other hand, I had followed the deepest feeling of connection that I had ever experienced. Was this to open me up to even more richness of life and realities? I was to realise that the connection was more with the land, rather than the distorted relationship. The land was, in fact, the driving force.

Ever the optimist and in amongst the emotional angst, the spark of light inside grew as I realised that this was still an opportunity and the door had well and truly opened. I remembered the unwavering connection I had with the islands of Hawaii. The reason I was attracted to going there in the first place, how I felt when I was there and how I yearned for knowledge. This wasn't a disaster, this was the perfect chance to really embrace and understand who it is that I am, to honour my journey in life and to follow my heart into truth. My meeting with Adam, was a blessing in disguise as it simply enabled me to let go of my past and to allow the flow of life to enter me again.

I was so grateful to be with Basho at that moment in time. "Basho, what am I going to do?" I said. I had a suitcase full of clothes, a stash of money, a few knick-knacks and photos of my family and friends. I realised staying in the UK was out of the question. My heart was still set on going to Hawaii.

Basho knew quite a few people who lived in Maui and he brilliantly came up with a plan. Talk about being in the right place at the right time. He called his long time friend in Maui to ask if he knew of anywhere I could lodge. Incredibly, Basho's friend said, "Our lodger has just moved out, we've just repainted the room and it's available, Jane could come and stay here." He said he wouldn't charge very much and when was I coming? No questions asked. It was a done deal. I had somewhere to stay. In the space of an hour, yet again my whole life did a flip! At this stage I still didn't know how I was going to survive. I had enough money to last me for a few months, but that was living with Adam. I trusted everything would be well and to me this was confirmation that I had to go. It seemed one door closed and another opened almost immediately.

I decided that I would go and make the most of it. There was no turning back. I wanted to find out why I had such a deep connection to Hawaii and why I kept on making the same 'mistakes,' so I would go and explore and find some answers. My decision to go was one of the best choices I ever made. The next few months were transformational as my perceptions were changed forever.

The day I left, Mum and Dad took me to the airport. It was a very emotional time. Mum cried and clung onto me for the first time ever. I balled my eyes out on the plane as I settled down for the transatlantic flight into a new reality. It was extremely tough to leave my parents at the airport. I didn't know if I would see them again, that's how it felt. But, I somehow felt liberated. Going into the unknown was exciting.

Getting off the plane in Maui and recognising the familiar smells and sounds made it all seem like this was the best thing I had ever done. I immediately felt at home. The warm air enveloped my body. I had no idea what to expect when I arrived. Basho's friends had given me a number to call when I got to Kahului airport. I called and Keith answered. He told me where to meet him and I duly went to find the car park where he was due to pick me up. He would be in a tree surgeon truck, whatever that looked like. Anyhow, the only truck to turn up was his.

He seemed pleasant and friendly, although I didn't quite understand everything he said! It always took me by surprise, the American language. Yes I know that sounds strange. What I mean is, although we speak English, it's not quite the same. Words are said in a different context and it took a while to adjust.

Keith had fair hair, blue eyes and was in his late forties. He was fit and casual looking as was everyone in Hawaii. He was a tree surgeon. We took a thirty minute ride to their home located on the south side of the island. Keith, and his wife Christine, lived in a single story four bedroom home, set in a residential area, one block from the ocean shore. They had a couple of other properties which they let out as holiday homes.

Christine was German, which was great as there was a familiarity to her. She was tall, blond with a slight lisp and very fit. We clicked straight away as she toured me around their lovely home and introduced me to all the idiosyncrasies of daily life. I was taken through the housekeeping rules and met Ben, a cuddly golden retriever. I was shown the fridge, which was absolutely full of healthy sprouts, beans, juices and an abundance of natural herbal tablets for all manner of complaints. Everything was tickety boo.

My room was small but comfortable and I was very grateful. There was another lodger in the house who had the bigger bedroom with its own patio and shower room. She had been there for three months and was waiting on her own house being ready to move into. Her name was Ella. She worked as a set designer on big Hollywood films. I was later to discover that every other Californian in Maui worked in films. Ella was very talented and spent her time in between films, teaching scuba diving on Maui. What an idyllic life! I would be moving into her room, once she had left.

Still unsure of what to do next, I settled down and took some time out to relax. I wanted some answers to my life. I realised a deep need for help, a bit like when I turned thirty and visited the doctor, not knowing what sort of help I needed, yet by going there the right help came my way. However, there were so many therapists and healers here it was daunting and didn't feel right just picking one out of the phone book. I sensed I needed something different. I would wait and bide my time and keep focussing on meeting the right type of person to help me. I felt strange and a little sad, away from my life back in the UK. It all felt surreal in this moment. I couldn't get Adam out of my mind. He was there all the time and I half wanted to bump into him.

After about a week, I was beginning to settle into a routine. You couldn't do anything but live a healthy lifestyle here. Fresh fruit, fresh clean air, just fresh everything actually. Christine and Keith were great and as we shared a mutual friend in Basho we got on famously. I'd started to jog in the morning along the ocean front. The water would be glistening in the early morning light and the gentle waves would break over the shoreline. The reality of where I was and what I had done beginning to kick in.

One morning, as I was doing some food shopping, I bumped into Adam. I couldn't believe it. I had been thinking I might like to see him again, but when it happened I wanted to run away. He looked good. We exchanged small talk and I asked him how his new girlfriend was. He just said,"Oh she wasn't right. It wasn't serious." Flabbergasted at his flippancy, I tried to stay cool, exchanged a little more small talk and said goodbye. He said, "See you around," and off I went. My legs were like jelly. I wasn't sure how I felt, was I angry?

For the next week I kept on bumping into Adam at different places and different times. My mind started going into overdrive. Maybe it's for a reason, maybe I'm meant to be with him and so it went on. My mind played tricks, as I realised I was really bereft and needy for love.

One day, after bumping into him again, he said, "This is ridiculous. Why don't we get together and give it another try?" My heart jumped a beat, without thinking I said, "Yes." We arranged to meet for an evening meal. He took me to one of the best hotels for a dinner at sunset. He hadn't changed, still a little aloof and self obsessed. He told me all about this girl, that had been the cause of so much upset, not just for me but for him as well it seemed. I couldn't believe he had been so frivolous about the whole thing. He continued to tell me his plans for the future. He wanted to give his acting career one last chance which meant a focus on himself.

In the meantime, I sat and listened. He really wasn't interested in me as a person at all, this was all about him. I should have walked away, but I didn't as my heart was aching.

He continued to talk and then said, "Well, if we are going to be together

I want an open relationship."

"What the hell does an open relationship mean?" I said!

"Well it might not happen, but I want the option of seeing other women."

I wasn't quick enough in my mind to respond and say, "Not on your life. We are past the dating stage."

I simply replied that I wasn't happy about this at all, but would give it a go. What was I doing? I realised that my self esteem was at rock bottom. I couldn't hold my own and I was completely vulnerable.

He had played me from the moment we met and I had allowed it. I'd given up everything for the dream of being in love and I had allowed him to break my heart, yet here I was allowing him back in again under his terms. What the hell was I doing!? My thoughts and feelings were totally at odds yet again. The reality of what was right for me and what was right for him were miles apart. Yet here I was agreeing to abide by his rules, albeit making it very plain that I was not happy with this and would back out at the first sign of any infidelity happening. I simply needed to get this man out of my hair!

I continued with this facade for about four weeks. As far as I am aware he never saw anyone else during this time as I would spend my nights at his place. He would be a completely different person at night to the one he became during the day, and I actually liked him again. However, daytime was about him, no one else. He was incredibly narcissistic in every way. Obsessed with his body and looks and playing the game. He treated me with disregard during the day. At night he would cuddle up and roles would change. He became soft and gentle and couldn't do enough for me. He was like a little boy needing some love and that's what kept me there.

Slowly, I came to my senses. I began to hate the way I was behaving. It wasn't going anywhere and I couldn't live with the fact that at anytime he could pull the plug, because the relationship was on his terms and my feelings and dreams didn't matter.

I started to get myself together and become aware again of this distortion I was living. I talked to him about finishing because I was getting very little from our relationship. My interest was definitely waning. Although I still really loved what seemed to be his vulnerability, he couldn't satisfy my needs in any way, shape or form so there was no mutual relationship. I plucked up the courage and decided to finish with him. When I told him, he laughed and didn't believe me at first, but I stayed away.

After about a week and a half he called me and asked me round for a chat. I gave in. It didn't take much did it? So we met, but I had strengthened in our time apart and I finally realised the reality and the depth of the distortion. There was a tremendous pull between us, but we wanted such different things and I wasn't interested anymore, he simply wasn't good enough for me.

So I left, telling him I didn't want to see him again and for a while I avoided going to the beach where we had first met. A few weeks later, after I thought it would be safe, I went down to the beach early in the day as I knew if he turned up it wouldn't be until after lunchtime. I enjoyed my swim and was just about to leave when he turned up much earlier than normal. It was strange and surreal as we ignored each other!

Then all of a sudden he came over and said, "You have to stop it."

I said, "I don't know what you mean?"

He didn't know either. It was very strange. When I saw him, all those initial feelings I held for him when we first met were prominent in my mind and I couldn't stop thinking about him. At some level he was picking up on the action of my thoughts and it disturbed him. I realised I had a responsibility to let him go completely on all levels. I recognised that the power of my thoughts and emotions was keeping us connected, with as much potency as a physical bond.

I stopped going back to that beach, or anywhere else where we had been together. As soon as I noticed I was thinking of him, I changed my thoughts and focussed on something else. I started going to daily Bikram yoga classes. An extreme form of yoga, practised in a hot room and I focussed on letting go of any physical, emotional and mental ties I held with him. I remembered how I felt back in the UK before I came, the real pull of me coming here, not because of Adam, but because of my connection with the land. There was no going back. I continued to stay open into finding someone who could help me with discovering what the connection to the islands was about.

Pathfinder

Another day in paradise. I stopped off at a health food store to pick up some supplies and glanced at the notice board outside. There was nothing much of interest, the normal adverts for therapists, healers, yoga teachers, workshops and the like. Then down tucked away in the corner of the board was a business card. It said Pathfinder and a name and number to call.

My heart jumped and I couldn't see anything else except this card, I walked away, but something pulled me back. I wrote down the number to call later in the day. I had no idea what a pathfinder was, but it struck a chord with me - another gut feeling. I eventually got through to a lovely lady and I liked what I heard. She sounded exactly what I was after, no airy fairy stuff, plain and simple getting to the truth. I arranged to see her for a consultation.

Nicole was half Hawaiian, tall, slim and blond. It had been acknowledged before birth that she would be a Kahuna and when born was given to her Hawaiian grandmother to be bought up to learn and embrace the ancient knowledge known as Huna. Her Hawaiian Grandmother passed on the ancient esoteric wisdom of the language and Nicole had developed her own particular skill of 'seeing' the truth as well as working with herbs and plants of the land.

This particular kind of Kahuna works through the transformation of the blueprint that we bring into this life, with all its baggage from previous lives. Most Kahunas are bringers of light and healing and can work on many different levels through the physical, mental, emotional and spiritual levels. They bring in a level of consciousness to shine light where there is darkness and confusion including past life distortions and karmic patterns. Being in their presence opens up the gateways so you can see, for yourself, the source of discomfort, caused by destructive patterns, behaviours and belief systems. Becoming more conscious allows for an opportunity to choose to change should you want to.

We continued with some healing sessions and then she mentioned that I might benefit by doing a real life journey. We would spend a day or two together, solely focussed on letting go of the 'clutter' that blocked my own growth and development. Getting to the truth of who I am. That's what I really wanted, to really get to know who I was, not what was expected of me, to understand that which I felt was missing. This is what I had come for.

I wanted to go get to the root of whatever it was I needed to get to the root of! I felt on a precipice again in my life, seeming to go from one disaster to another, particularly in relationships, just about keeping my head above water. I was doing reasonably well in my professional work, but never really achieving greatness, I felt weighed down with so much emotional insecurity and baggage that didn't seem necessary anymore. Although I had already done an awful lot of work in healing the wounds that I carried, I somehow knew this would go really deep and was essential for living the life that I wanted. I needed to get to the next level and I hadn't gone through all that pain to get here for nothing!

My birthday was due and we were to meet up early on my birthday for a two day trip. I was to pack for an overnight stay. The week before I had missed my period, didn't think anything of it and put it down to the change of being in a different country, new environment, however I began to wonder.

I had been told a few years before that I would never have children. I was diagnosed with polycystic ovary syndrome, although this diagnosis was disputed years later. This had come about when I gave up on taking the contraceptive pill years before when I ran out of them in Madeira. I had decided that it was a good a time to stop so I did.

I never liked taking the pill anyway as it seemed to me to go against Mother Nature. I knew I would suffer heavy painful periods and get really bloated every month if I stopped, but I couldn't go on any longer with this conflict inside. After I gave up taking the pill, I had horrible symptoms. I would get cold sweats; I put on weight, had spots all over my face and generally felt awful. I decided this didn't seem normal, so went off to get checked out.

I was back in the UK at this time and appallingly treated. There was very little care or sensitivity from the health professionals and absolutely no help or support forthcoming. They gave me a diagnosis and promptly left me out to dry to cope on my own. I was told that because I wasn't in a relationship or married, they weren't prepared to give me the operation that was required and bluntly told me that I would never conceive and that was it. I was left feeling angry and upset at the lack of sensitivity. The symptoms were challenging enough, surely there must be some help and support. It was a painful experience as I grieved for the fact that I could not have children. I felt that I shouldn't have something like this. I was fit and healthy and it didn't feel right.

With the pent up anger at how I felt being ostracised because I was unmarried and single, at least that's what it felt like to me, I wasn't going to let this destroy my life and I certainly wasn't going to go back on the pill as they had suggested. I had already made it clear that it didn't suit me. The thought of having to change the pill every six to twelve months and sometimes longer, because I would develop unwanted symptoms, simply wasn't good enough for me to renege. I decided to research the condition myself and I made some changes in my life.

I realised I could balance my hormones myself through cleansing my system. This was before I had trained to become a Polarity Therapist. I took some advice from a nutritionist and I simply went back to basics. I ate fruit and vegetables and cut out milk, wheat, alcohol and caffeine. I felt great and never had a reoccurrence of the symptoms, so now I eat whatever I feel like eating. However, the pain of being told so bluntly that I would never have children had stayed with me. It took the best part of six months to get into a reasonable balance and it wasn't easy.

Miracle

So, here I was in Hawaii, my period late and beginning to wonder what if? The day before my birthday I bought a pregnancy test and found out I was pregnant. It must have been an immaculate conception because my time with Adam wasn't exactly a successful sexual relationship. I was in deep, deep shock. Never in a million years would I ever see myself pregnant. Many times I wanted to believe that I would make a great Mum, but couldn't bear the thought of even contemplating the possibility, knowing that it wasn't possible.

A waterfall of tumbling thoughts and feelings flooded me." What should I do? I'm no spring chicken...... I'll have to get rid of it..... Oh no, I couldn't do that........ It's a life, how amazing I'm going to have a baby!.... Oh what joy........Oh what trauma......What will my parents think!? What will Adam think?.....Where will I have it?......... How am I going to look after the baby?... Where will I live?.... How will I cope?" Panic! I couldn't say anything to Keith and Christine. I had to be sure first. "What are they going to think?...... I'll have to find somewhere else to live.... I don't want to go home," and so on. The mind and emotions took over with many questions and not many answers.

I felt like I had done something wrong and that it was wrong for me to be having a baby. I felt like everyone would disapprove. I'm not married, not even living with the father. What a disgrace. I felt like a girl in trouble and felt like I would be highly disapproved of. Where did all this come from?

Thank God for Nicole. The morning of my birthday I got up and I realised now that I could see that my body was changing. No wonder I had been feeling tired. Nicole came in with the biggest bunch of yellow roses, the exact number representing my age, and a huge smile! I told her I had something to say before we started on our trip. "I am pregnant," I said. She was shocked, said she hadn't seen it, (they see what they are meant to see), but then very genuinely she gave me the biggest hug and said she was so happy for me. It made me cry. The first person that I had told was completely supportive and joyful about the whole scenario and it felt the most natural thing to happen. I thought I would get disapproval, however her reaction set me free. The feelings of disapproval and disgust went immediately out of the window.

For the first time I felt relieved and very, very excited. I was going to be alright, no one could take away this feeling of joy. The next two days of my real life journey were gentle and exactly what I needed. The journeys takes the form of going within, visiting special sacred areas on the land (portals) that raise the vibration so you can become conscious of long standing patterns and distortions. This is done through meditations and visualisation that create a conscious connection from the unknown to the known. Healing takes place at a deep neurological level once the light shines in and is supported by the ancient knowledge of our ancestors and is supported by the high vibration of the islands known as Hawaii.

My journey took me into infinite possibilities and released and broke some old very destructive belief patterns and behaviours. I was breaking new waters, into a new enlightened perspective on my life so far.

THE BIG SURF

"There are no classes in life for beginners: right away you are always asked to deal with what is most difficult"
Rainer Maria Rilke

Visions from the past

It was day one of my real life journey. We started with a good breakfast and set off in Nicole's jeep towards the back side of the now dormant volcano Haleakala. On our drive towards the barren side of the island, we saw an owl flying over our vehicle, an unusual sighting in the daytime. Everywhere dragonflies danced and all manner of animals came into view, pheasants, chickens and goats. The place was full of vibrancy and aliveness. I began to become aware of my feelings much more than normal. I sensed things stirring inside again.

We came to a place where the road became a track and we slowed down. It was an eerie site. There were long slopes of ancient volcanic lava rock, jagged, pointed and dark, peppered with green patches of shrubbery and the odd tree. The lava field created a dramatic backdrop to the deep blue ocean. It was silent and still. We stopped and got out of the jeep. There was a wall of rocks close to where we stood.

Nicole asked me to tune in and to get a sense of what was going on for me in this moment. The theme of the feelings and pictures that flashed through my mind was of controlling, manipulative energy that created pain and hurt in my life and lack of self-worth. It was vividly clear. I was amazed at the clarity. This was to set the foundation for the work of releasing that needed to be done over the next couple of days.

Nicole chanted and we sat quietly tuning into the surrounding energies. I felt a sudden shift and a clearing in my mind. The feelings of pain and hurt lifted and a strong sense of protection prevailed around me. It felt like a preparation and bought in a presence that enabled me to be in the moment with what was happening and to feel secure. We gave thanks and drove on.

We lunched in Kula and drove down towards La Parouse Bay. During this time I was encouraged to talk about my life as a child and my relationship with my sister and parents. We ended up in an ancient village site where families once lived on the volcanic rock. La Parouse is set in a beautiful sheltered bay, where dolphins come and play early in the mornings. To the right of the area is a stunning smaller bay, almost a pond, with white sand giving a dramatic contrast to the surrounding black rocks. The ocean was turquoise blue.

There were two loose rocks, big enough to sit on, side by side – male and female. We sat and connected with our surroundings. I closed my eyes and watched the visions come into my mind. I saw big Hawaiian women, dressed in a traditional way. All of them were happy and laughing, sitting making tapa cloths and headdresses and leis. It was a picture of women together enjoying life, mothers, sisters, aunts and nieces. In my minds' eye I was invited to sit with them. They were so loving it felt an honour to be in their presence. I felt happy and loved. They were all very excited about the baby on the way, and I saw them telling me what to do and although I couldn't hear their words, I sensed what they were saying. Eat well, rest a lot and we are here to support you.

I slowly opened my eyes just in time to see the sky turn a soft orange. Tears of joy seeped from my eyes. I felt a strong sense of nurturing support surrounding me. Everything seemed to confirm that it was perfectly alright that I was with baby and I was going to be a mother. I had never felt that sense of nurture or safety from my own mother. This was such a blessing, it allowed me to feel what it was like to receive such a love and showed me how I could be with my own child. The vision allowed me to recognise that which I was missing in my own childhood, not just for me but for my siblings as well. It was an opportunity to feel the depth of nurture and safety that a mothers' love can give and, actually, that I had experienced this before in previous lifetimes. Whatever karma was being played out in our particular family, it was now important for me to let go of all the hurt, manipulation and emotional confusion surrounding this current life adventure. I may have missed out this time, but I have experienced this kind of love before and its time to heal the wounds and forgive. I was able to really forgive my sister and my mother and although there is a residue or reminder in the reality of my daily life, I can truly see them in their higher light and it no longer affects me. When I feel unwanted or unsafe, I simply reconnect with this deeper knowing of female love and affection that is always there.

Nicole closed the session for the day, thanking the animals and all our spirit guides for their guidance. I left a lei as an offering to the Hawaiian ladies of La Parouse and we drove off to our hotel for the night.

Quality of value

As a treat for my birthday, we stayed in the Grand Wailea, a very posh hotel indeed. Our room was amazing. Nicole ran a bath for me with candles, aromatherapy oils and petals. I felt like a princess and very well taken care of, continuing the theme of the day. I'd not experienced this level of care for a very long time and it was lovely. My experience during the day, and the way Nicole was looking after me, left me with a feeling of a deep mother's love and nurture. There was no judgement about my condition, just complete support.

We dressed up and went out for a lovely dinner in a beach restaurant. Nicole gave me a gift. It was a beautiful necklace with a stunning green peridot stone as the centre piece. I felt very special. The last time someone bought me something special was my ex husband when we first got together.

I was learning again what it was like to be cared for. I slept peacefully and dreamt of my womb getting stronger to hold the baby and I dreamt of a figurine, a dream I've had before. Normally in this dream the figurine would be in a circle, but this time it was on its own, something had changed. I woke up feeling tired yet relaxed and with a renewed sense of wanting to really look after my physical body and slightly worried that I had been doing too an intense form of yoga, not knowing that I was pregnant. I hoped this hadn't damaged the baby in any way. I decided I would stop immediately.

Whilst I waited for Nicole, I sat and meditated for a while on the balcony, looking out onto a glistening ocean. After a scrumptious breakfast of tropical fruits and eggs, my second day of journeying started. It was another day of shedding negative, manipulative and controlling energy. We drove to Paia, a rather funky, alternative town on the north shore which is a hangout for surfers and the like. We did a little window shopping, and normally I would browse quickly, thinking I didn't need anything and why would I waste time buying something for myself, so I won't bother to look properly.

In that moment I recognised that I didn't value myself at all. Why not see the value of things and why am I not worthy of looking at the value? It was a wake up call and made me recognise that I am worthy of quality and value, just like everyone else. So, I started to think and feel in those terms; of me being valued and worthy of greatness. In turn, I felt special inside. Since then, I've been able to draw on that feeling and immediately any old unhealthy feelings subside and go.

We continued on our journey, this time up towards the north west of the island where tucked away on a hilltop overlooking the Wailuku region was a beautiful Heiau called Kukuipuka Heiau – a place of healing and refuge. It was well kept and divinely peaceful. As we entered this sacred area, I felt like I was surrounded with a soft supportive feminine energy again. I walked around and when I felt drawn to a stone I sat with it, tuned in and felt and sensed what emerged. In Hawaii, everything has a soul or energy, rather like the stones back in Portland that held a particular essence.

The Heiau was a square space marked out with ancient stones, all different and unique and each with a story to tell. I felt drawn to sit against one of them. I sat with this stone for a while and a sense of the purity of connection flowed through me from heaven to earth and gave me strength.

I then moved to another stone. As I sat, I sensed a quality of transformation which was much more energetic in its essence. Then a vision emerged. There was a butterfly fluttering around then, all of a sudden, it changed into a murderous picture. A tourmaline ocean, carrying what looked like a Tahitian long boat, full of warriors. The boat beached and the warriors ran through a village, killing the women and children. I lost the vision as it was very disturbing. After I gathered myself together I asked to replay the scene. It had changed. This time I saw a protective white barrier against the warriors coming ashore and the outcome was different as the village was defended by an intangible force. I felt such power, love and gratefulness as the scene played out and lives were spared. I thanked the stone for its message, even though I didn't entirely understand it at the time, but I guessed it was from a past life and moved to another stone.

Finally, there was one more stone that I felt drawn to sit with. As I closed my eyes, I saw were three elements to the scene; a delicate flower; a black energy that turned to white and a birdman figure overseeing the whole. I felt like I was seeing three aspects of myself in a way that I didn't quite understand at this moment in time.

When I think back to these images, they seemed like scenes out of a movie. I felt incredibly grateful to be able to see, just by simply sitting, quietening the mind and connecting into what was around me. The scenes gave me insight into the past and the future both in symbolic terms and in reality. The energy of the land and its people lends itself to help heal the deep seated wounds that we carry around with us like extra baggage into future lives unless we choose to wake up and do something about it. Like other sacred areas around the world, this profound land of light was giving me an opportunity to open up to different levels of consciousness, as the veil in the Islands is very thin. We are not alone.

We finished the two days with a slap up meal. I was very tired and this was just the ticket. I got back to my lodgings and immediately felt that I was under attack. I had told Keith and Christine that I would be away for two nights. The questions started. Where had I been? What had I been doing? I felt like I was being interrogated! I retreated to my room for the evening and didn't surface until the next morning. Christine had already gone to work when I got up in the morning, thankfully, and Keith just asked how I was. He said I looked different. They had obviously sensed something was changing with me. Perhaps it was a little scary.

Spending the last two days with Nicole had raised my vibration to allow me to see even more clearly. I had fully accepted my position and realised the power of a mother's love. I felt a lot lighter as the heaviness of unhealthy family related patterns and manipulative energies that I had allowed to batter me around in life had, on one level, released and gone. However, I felt there was much more to do. I found Christine and Keith's reaction on my return interesting. A new strength had emerged.

Responsibility

Now back to the practicalities of life. I had to decide on when to tell Keith and Christine about the baby. I felt obliged to tell them as I am sure they would notice something different soon and I was excited now, incredibly excited, and I really wanted to share this with someone. Adam, I guessed, wouldn't want to know as he had since found another girlfriend. I had seen them together in the car one day, but, of course,

I felt I had an obligation to tell him as the father. He may want to be in the child's life.

As I started to think about the reality again, I became nervous about the whole thing. Doubts started to crowd in. How would I support the baby? I'd have to go back to the UK. How could I cope being a single Mum? There were so many questions to answer. I was sure about one thing; no one was going to tell me what I should or shouldn't do. Most of my early life there was always someone telling me they knew better about what was best for me. Not any more, it would be my decision as to what I did with the baby and my life from now on. I had gained a renewed strength and confidence and I sensed that anything was possible.

I went to get checked out at the clinic. They took all the tests and gave me the necessary information I needed. All was going well. I became really tired and lethargic and felt obliged to say something soon as I wanted to share my news with someone at least.

Keith and Christine asked me one evening to eat with them and watch a movie. During the meal they started asking questions, so it sort of slipped out that I was going to have a baby. Christine went into overdrive. They were both so excited. I never expected this reaction.

The next day, Christine came into my room and said she wanted to talk to me. I knew that she had always wanted a child but Keith didn't. She was a similar age to me and this must have hurt her. However, she said she and Keith had talked about this and they wanted to support me fully in whatever way they could. They would help me raise the baby and help me somehow get a work permit. They had a couple of properties and offered me a cottage to rent. It all sounded perfect for them.

I said I would think seriously about their offer however, it was early days and I still hadn't told anyone else and needed to get my head straight first. Next on the list was to tell my parents. Oh my God, I wondered what their reaction was going to be. I'm thousands of miles away and their youngest is calling to tell them she is up the duff! I felt like a little girl again having done something wrong.

I finally called them.

"Hi, Mum, Dad, I'm going to have a baby"

"Oh Janie are you?" Mum said.

Dad laughed. "You're going to have a baby"?

Mum said how wonderful. I was so surprised about their reaction. Then the questions came. "Are you going to marry the father?"

Dad said, "Well he is going to have to support you both."

"Where will you live?" And so on.

I just said very calmly, "Everything is in hand. The father will know in due course, when I am ready to tell him and don't worry about a thing, I am in good hands and in a good place."

They both said they were happy for me. It was just the best thing that could happen to me, but I do need to get married! Phew. It was done.

I then told my friend Basho. He was so excited and also wanted to help me raise the child. What great friends I have, but there was a price as I realised the responsibility of this whole scenario. Everyone seemed to have their own agenda. It was a volatile situation. Personal dramas were playing out through my actions and life choices. I should have kept quiet as I began to realise the enormity of my actions and how it seemed to affect those nearest to me, but I was so excited and I wanted to share my joy.

I spent the next few weeks, enjoying the feelings in my body, as it began to change shape. I became protective about myself. I really thought about what I was putting in my body and generally slept when I felt like it, which was a lot. I ate when I felt like it and tried to stay away from being with people who had there own opinions and agenda. I was also feeling very fragile and vulnerable. I had been offered some part time casual work, which gave me a small income and I was still okay for money too, so that was one less thing to think about.

I needed to get away from the lodging situation as it was becoming stifling, I couldn't do anything without being asked what I was doing, where I was going, what I was eating. It was like being a child again! It was the hardest thing to tell them I was moving out into an apartment down the road, for my own space and to give them back their privacy. As it turned out, it worked out really well for us. The relationship balanced out and I became their friend rather than a child living in their house and I was invited round for dinner and to watch movies, which was much healthier.

Out of the blue

I checked my emails on a regular basis and out of the blue I received an email from Gerry, the guy from the Lomi course whom I had quite liked. He was coming to Maui for a break and had heard I was on the island. Would I be interested in meeting up with him? Now I didn't know if he knew the situation I was in. Of course, I would love to meet up with him but I was a little worried about his expectation.

We met at his hotel for lunch and it was great to see him. I was fairly emotional and sensitive with hormonal changes and tired all the time. We caught up with all the latest news and then I told him my news. He looked upset. Then he explained why he had come. He had met a girl from Europe, yet he was unsure as to whether or not to commit to her. Gerry had come for a break as it seemed he was at a cross roads himself. He came to explore if there was any possibility for us to be partners, as he had felt a connection on the course and thought we might be good together. He said he was ready to have a family and to settle down.

I was truly taken aback. I had no idea how he felt about me and what timing! Here was a great guy, a real catch, sat telling me he wanted what I wanted. Had I screwed up somewhere along the line in my choices!? But, it was a non starter right now and we would have been together for all the wrong reasons, in my eyes we didn't know each other at all.

I really wasn't in a good space to consider a relationship with anyone. I couldn't have coped and I had nothing of myself to offer him at that moment in time and I didn't feel the same way about him as I was too engrossed in what was going on in my body and thinking of how to sort my life out. He offered to support and take care of the baby with me and made it very clear that he wanted more children.

I was in my early forties and it scared me to even think about having more. I was still getting used to the fact that I had actually conceived. It was a real shame. I shall never forget the sadness, but I was empty and simply had nothing left for him. I felt his pain. I know he stayed on an extra week and after that he left and I never heard from him again. If he had turned up just a few weeks later, it could have been entirely different.

Confrontation

My apartment became my sanctuary and a great space to think and feel clearly. Still unsure how and when to tell Adam, I was frightened about his reaction for some reason, perhaps it was the thought of rejection and disapproval. One day I plucked up the courage to call him. It was very nerve racking. I had planned in my head what to say, but it didn't quite go to plan, as he demanded to know why I wanted to see him. I'm not a very good at concealing the truth and couldn't think of an excuse that would be credible, so I plunged in and told him I was pregnant with his baby. The first thing he said was, "Are you sure and are you sure its mine?" which really pissed me off, as I certainly am not able to cope with being involved with more than one person at a time! After he realised I was serious, he agreed to meet over a meal and he said, "I'll call you in the next couple of days to arrange it." I didn't hear from him for a week and by this time I was getting really annoyed at his lack of sincerity. It seemed he really wasn't bothered. I wanted to know how he saw his level of involvement with the child, if any, so I could start to make plans as to where I needed to be.

I called him instead and arranged for him to come to me at my apartment. Whether he liked it or not he was the father of the child. I set the scene, got fresh flowers and lit a candle as a form of protection for me. He bowled up in his arrogant way, sat straight down in a chair, and I asked him if he wanted to be involved in the child's upbringing. He immediately went on the defensive and a whole load of nasty comments came out of his mouth.

Without any prompting he said, "I would never marry you and I don't want any involvement with the baby."

I knew he already had one child and was experiencing difficulties with his little girl wanting to have both parents together, so was not surprised when he said would not want to go through that again. Then he said,"You'll be on your own raising it. Do you know how difficult it is to raise a child on your own? Wouldn't it be best for you to have a termination? Think about your age, you're not a youngster anymore."

Inside I was ready to burst out in tears. This really hurt but I held it together. I had expected this kind of reaction, knowing the person he was. Then came the icing on the cake,

"Who have you told?"

"Why," I asked

"I have a new girlfriend and I don't want her knowing, as she is important to me."

Feeling very small, I mumbled something about not to worry, the secret is safe. No one would know in his social circle.

I had expected a negative response, understandably he must have been fearful, but it really flagged up to me how little he knew about the person I was. I truly wasn't expecting anything from him. I certainly would never want to be with this man, let alone marry him. He was arrogant and a bully, completely insensitive and without compassion for anyone else's feelings.

I knew on one level that he didn't believe me. I guess our meeting lasted all of twenty minutes or so. I told him I would be having the baby, as I would never consider terminating a gift of life and clarified his words that he didn't want any involvement. That was it! I let him out of the apartment and out of my life for good. He turned round at the door and put his hand on my belly and laughed, as if he was secretly pleased, kissed me on the cheek and said, "Look after yourself."

I closed the door and fell to the ground. I felt like I had been stabbed in the stomach with a knife. I held onto the baby for dear life, as it felt like my whole existence was breaking apart. My tears were like a day of big surf, they kept on coming and bursting out, gut wrenching, so deep it hurt. It all seemed such an unusually powerful response. My baby must have felt rejected.

A dark place

It seemed like an age before I finally got myself together. I went to the kitchen to get a glass of water and the glass broke in my hands. Something was broken. I began to worrying about the impact of my emotional outburst on the baby. It focussed me on how I was going to proceed from here. I had decided that perhaps I should go back to the UK, as I had no means of earning a lot of money here, not unless I had investment for a business. By going back to the UK now I could come back here later to have the baby. I knew I would have a lot of support here. Families don't necessarily mean blood relatives in Hawaiian culture. I knew that I and the baby would be supported anytime I came back.

I began to feel very unwell. I felt extremely tired, and then I got a dull ache in my lower abdomen. I went to the doctors for a check up. He said everything was fine but if the pain continued, to come back. Two days later I was in excruciating pain and was losing some blood. I really didn't want to bother Christine and Keith. In any case they were at work and Nicole was overseas. So I drove myself across the island to the emergency unit of the hospital.

I was checked out and told I may be having a miscarriage. I had a scan which was agonising as it seemed an age before the technician said anything. I knew something was up. There was no heartbeat. I was sent home and told to expect the worst. The miscarriage would happen over the next couple of days, and if it didn't, I was to come back.

Later the next day I lost the baby. I was devastated and stayed in my apartment for a couple of days, fending off telephone calls from work, saying I was tired. I drove to the doctor for a check up to make sure everything had cleared. It was an incredibly sad time. I was in a very dark, despairing place. The life was sucked out of me it all seemed, deeply sorrowful.

Finally, I went round to see Christine and Keith and told them the news. They were also very upset and incredibly supportive and continued to be until I left. I felt so sorry for Christine as she was so looking forward to helping me, not able to have a child herself. I then had to tell everyone who I had told and that was equally tough.

I look back on that time now and it seemed the turning point in the pregnancy was when Adam effectively rejected us both. Something inside me died. It was nothing to do with a relationship with Adam, apart from the fact that we had created this situation, it was deeper than that, somehow the whole thing seemed like another lifetime. Like the vision I had before at Kukuipuka Heiau with the women of a village being raped and murdered by warriors. This time though it was more representative of male energy and its potential destructive power over female energy if boundaries are not in place. I had learned that anything is possible in life, even when experts tell you something is not possible. Never say never. I actually felt blessed to have experienced a tiny bit of motherhood.

The next couple of weeks I spent in a daze. My body hurt, my heart hurt and I was desperately trying to make sense of it all. My flight back to the UK was looming but even after everything that had happened, I really didn't want to go back. I changed my flight to leave on the day my visa ran out, to get the maximum time on the island and decided to do another 'journey' with Nicole. There was a lot more to clear out. Before that it was Thanksgiving and I was invited to Nicole's home to be with her family for the day. That was a very special time. I felt love all around. We shared great food and great conversation and lots of laughter and real sense of normal family life. It was light relief from the despair that I felt inside.

Dolphin magic

Following Thanksgiving, I visited all my favourite places, for solace and healing and, on a beautiful afternoon, I took a trip to La Parouse, a special place of memories which happened to be a dolphin haven. I arrived and immediately bumped into someone I knew. Paula had given me a Polarity treatment the first time I was in Maui a year earlier. She was about the same age as me and she could see I was upset. As I knew her, I told her I had just had a miscarriage. Unbelievably, she told me she was pregnant herself. I thought this can't be real, what on earth is going on here? She said because of her age, she had some complications and was here for some healing to help her through. There was a group of women who were developing a practise to solely focus on pregnancy through a form of cranial sacral healing in water. She asked me if I would like to receive some healing as well as she thought they wouldn't mind.

It was a true gift that I went there that afternoon. Two lovely women and one man, held me in the warm water of the lagoon and supported my body as the healing session evolved. I drifted off and I saw a vision of dolphins coming right into the shallow pond where we were. I received a very clear message that the dolphins were there for me, that the soul of the baby was okay and very strong, but the soul of the baby was worried about me. The grief was immense, I had to let go.

I surrendered to this whole scenario, didn't have any energy left and as I did so I felt an enormous wave of peace and pure light wash over me. I didn't feel the girls supporting me anymore; something else had taken over, just a sense of being suspended in light. I felt such love in that moment, it was overwhelming.

I gently came around and sat on my special rocks as they wrapped me in towels and blankets. I stayed until sunset, suspended in time, feeling clearer, lighter and stronger, ready to take on my next real life journey with Nicole.

The synchronicities of life become really strong, the more open we become to other possibilities. You never know how, one day, the connections and chance meetings can affect you. This meeting was truly a blessing.

Journey of lifetimes

It was a very different morning for my second real life journey. I drove towards Nicole's house on the cooler, wetter side of up country Maui. The morning was cloudy as I stopped outside her house. A deep foreboding struck me, as this time I didn't have the baby to nurture and protect, it was just me again and I began to feel very strange indeed.

We set off in the jeep. I had packed an overnight bag and bought along offerings for our journey. First stop breakfast. I had learned to always eat well during any healing process. As we travelled south towards the lava fields, a different way to last time, the sun had disappeared and a cloak of mist had come down from the mountain. It was eerie. Every now and then the cloud would break and we'd get an idea of where we were and I saw an owl and dragonflies again, a sure sign that we were not alone. Suddenly we broke free of the mist and stopped at a point with views over the ocean. Lava fields flowed down towards the water.

We sat quietly for a while, listening and watching and going within. I closed my eyes and images and feelings of all of the men in my life flashed before my eyes. All seemingly similar. Nicole opened the session with a prayer and a chant. After the opening ceremony, I was asked to pick up a stone that I felt drawn to. I chose a jagged piece of a'a lava rock*. As I held the rock, a strong, mellow male energy source seemed to surround me. It was light and powerful. The rock emanated a feeling of strength, warmth, vibrancy and expansion. For me it represented protection. I still hold it to this day when I need to. It became one of three rocks I was to keep and treasure from this journey. Then I heard a message in my head to get my eyes checked out – weird I thought.

We continued on and I became very aware of the changing energy outside of the car. Every area seemed to hold a story. I felt very small. We drove through one particular area of trees, I wound down the windows and Nicole asked me how it felt to me. I sensed it was a very deep, dark area that would either be your friend or foe. These interludes were all lessons, getting me used to tuning in to what's going on around and within, sensing the many dimensions that are present to us in every waking moment, sometimes relevant to our own individuality or global reality, sometimes not. We moved on. During the drive Nicole would ask me to talk about aspects of my relationships and more about my experiences in life so far. All this was preparing me for what was to come.

Hardly meeting anyone on the road, we finally came to the start of an area at the back of a place called Hana. The scenery had transformed from a barren land into lush greens and yellows. Stopping at a fruit stall to get some papaya, I began to feel really weird. My eyesight was going. I said to Nicole, "What's happening, my eye sight is going?" She just said, "Stay with it Jane. Keep holding onto the light." I didn't recognise the significance in that moment but I remembered the message from earlier on, which said to get my eyes tested and now I knew why. It seemed I was losing my sight!

On we drove. The further we went, the more my eyesight deteriorated. It was like a veil clouding my vision. It was scary to say the least, but there was nothing I could do, except pray that it would return. We reached a place called Koki beach, where we parked on the cliff top overlooking a craggy set of remote rocks in the distance, called Alau Island. Here we sat and ate some sandwiches and fruit. I was quiet and pensive and worried about my sight. Nicole was quiet and intense as if something big was about to happen. After eating, we sat just on the edge of the cliff. Birds were flying around the rocks in the distance. It was a dramatic scene. The sea was grey and waves were in turmoil and the sky thunderous. Something was happening to me. I had lost any clarity in my vision and I felt that I had become grey and misty like the weather. I remembered a similar experience back in 'Iao Valley when my sight was distorted, but this was much, much darker.

Nicole asked me how I was doing, I said, "Struggling. Why is my eyesight going?" All she said was, "Stay with it and focus on what you see and feel." So I did. It seemed as if I was experiencing life in greyness, not really living and not really dying. The feeling and thoughts became so strong. The indecisions and lack of my own worthiness and value in the relationships I had experienced and going against my gut instinct was how my whole life had been. I was being tossed around in life by situations and by those people around me and many times it felt like I should just die. In that moment in time, life was tough in my world. What was the point in living? Negative thoughts and feelings flowed through me. I didn't seem to be successful according to normal society. I wasn't married with children. I did not have a house and lots of other things. I had given up all that in search of a greater meaning for my life. The awfulness and emptiness I felt deep within was like rising surf rearing its ugly head.

I noticed through my blurred vision that birds were flying around in the distance over the isolated craggy rock. Again, it was very much representative of life on the edge, living and dying as a continuous process. After a while, during this eruption of emotions, thoughts and feelings, Nicole asked me to tune into a feeling of falling off the cliff. I found that difficult.

We sat for quite a while and I had my eyes closed. Then, suddenly, as if an unconscious part of me had made a decision, I saw an element of myself fall off the cliff! It was surreal. I opened my eyes then noticed a large piece of wood that was being battered by the waves in the ocean, one minute being beached the next just taken a little way out and then being battered back in again. It had no chance. I saw that piece of wood as a floundering victim, representative of my life. A question emerged in my mind. "What do you choose Jane?" I focussed all my attention as best that I could on the wood. Then something amazing happened, the wood began to find its place in the ocean. No longer was it being buffeted into land. It was almost like it had a mind of its own and it made its way back out into the ocean on a mission, sturdy and strong.

I realised that by letting go of a part of me that had been in the grey, I had allowed myself to become strong and vibrant in life again. The log represented and showed me that was happening. I had the power and the choice to change my reality. No one else did.

My eyesight got better immediately and clarity returned. I had made a choice to live life. I would have to work on that for a while longer, as the physical reality and daily patterns of life would have to catch up with the change in my blueprint, but what a relief I could see clearly again. It had been a tough day, very dark and I was exhausted.

The battle for my life

It had been raining heavily over the past few days, everything was sodden and damp, but now through the clouds the sun shone through and everything looked much brighter. The colours were deep and waterfalls vibrant with energy.

We drove into our hotel which was surrounded by lush tropical jungle and a complete contrast to the shiny bright resort hotels of the south coast. My mood was sombre. I was tired, I mean really tired. We rested and then in the hotel room we started more clearing processes.

I wrote down on bits of paper any word or sentence from people or situations that made me feel angry or awful at any time in my life. I sat for what seemed like hours writing words and sentences that made me feel this way. There was so much coming out. All the dodgy situations I had experienced, people who had hurt me physically, mentally and emotionally from family, friends and acquaintances, the whole lot. Anger against myself for allowing these situations was all coming up to the surface like a volcano. I felt wretched.

When the flow stopped, I read out each word or sentence and that was even tougher. I then folded the pieces of paper and put them into a silver bucket. We had candles burning around the room as outside it was getting dark. Night was drawing in. I lit a match and set fire to the paper in the bucket. The smoke was black. We closed the session leaving the ashes in the bucket to be ceremoniously washed away the next day.

After a warming bath, we got ready to go out for dinner in the hotel. It was a light relief from the heaviness of the day. We returned to sleep for a night that I will never forget. It was the darkest night I can ever remember. The room was heavy and I was in the bed nearest the shuttered window, the darkest part of the room. Only the glow of a candle left alight in the lounge area of our room was visible.

As soon as my eyes closed and my head hit the pillow, it was like a horror movie playing in a dream. I wasn't really asleep. Transfixed and frozen I watched as many horrible visions of creatures, beings, murderous angry scenarios played out in front of me. I couldn't sleep. All I could think of doing was focus on bringing in the light. I had been warned, that no matter how tough it was going to get, to keep focussing on the light and not to turn my back on anything that comes; equally not to engage, but hold firm to the light.

I understood why now. If I had turned and run, I would forever be followed and battered by life, just like the log in the ocean. If I engaged, I would become just like the horrible energies that were coming forth. If I stayed centred I would survive and live.

So as the night continued, I began to feel tired and weak from this constant bombardment

In the darkness I heard Nicole say to me, "How are you doing?"

"It's horrible and I'm struggling" I said.

"I know," she said, "Jane, just keep bringing in the light."

It was all the encouragement I needed. A renewed sense of determination flowed over me and I stood my ground. The last vision I had was of a black dark half monster, half horse, with flaring nostrils and an evil look coming towards me. It changed into two white beautiful horses that came galloping before me. Suddenly it all stopped, and surrounded in light, I fell into a deep heavy peaceful sleep.

Morning came and we woke early. We were going somewhere before breakfast. I was to wear a bathing costume and bring a towel. Off we went. It wasn't far. We parked up and walked down a path through spiders cobwebs with mosquitoes buzzing all around. Down we went until we came to a pond of water and an ominous looking cave. This looked scary! "What now," I thought! I was given instructions of what to do.

I got into the water. There was a natural barrier of rocks and debris blocking the entrance to the cave. The cave was black so you couldn't see in. I thought about all the negative thoughts, emotions and actions that had come up over the past months, years and lifetimes and let go of the key elements of these as best I could outside of the cave. I was letting go of my old life. Then I clambered over the barrier into the darkness. Under my feet I felt smooth stones. I couldn't see a thing as I waded into darkness and found a ledge to sit on. Once in the cave I started to only think positive thoughts about my life now and how I wanted to feel and be in the future. Slowly my breathing quietened and I found my self feeling nurtured and surrounded by a deep motherly energy. It felt like I was in a womb. All of a sudden, my eyes cleared. I could see clearly through the water. I saw the stones I was standing on, the shape of the cave. There was no light coming in, this was a different kind of light.

At the top left of the cave, it was slightly lighter. The walls were a brown, red grey colour and the rocks and stones at the bottom of the water were the same. I could see clearly and I was no longer scared. I felt an enormous sense of love and support. I sat for a while basking in this wonderful strength, gave thanks and climbed out into bright sunshine and vibrant colour.

I felt like a new born baby. Nicole wrapped me in towels and we took a slow walk back up to the car, and then back to the hotel, where I enjoyed lovely warm shower followed by a scrumptious breakfast. I didn't have many words. It all felt real, yet also surreal.

Slowly, as we drove back, the enormity of what I had just experienced began to seep into my consciousness. I was no longer afraid, yet feeling extremely fragile and vulnerable, really like a fledgling bird about to learn to fly. I felt totally cleansed.

I only had three days left before flying back to the UK. I spent that time quietly, visiting and meditating in my favourite places and gathering strength to help with the journey back. There was one particular meditation where an unusual scene played itself out. I saw a mountain peak with snow and a mountain peak dry and barren, then the ocean and a huge wave. I didn't realise at the time that this poignant vision was to come true the very next year

I enjoyed a meal with Nicole and her girls on the evening of my flight. It was incredibly difficult to say goodbye. They had become my family, but somehow I knew that I would be back, knowing that there are no limits and anything is possible. On both stages of my return flight I had a spare seat next to me, what a god send, it meant I had time and space to be and rest.

When lava cools forms a myriad of different shapes and types of lava. There are two main types of lava pahoehoe (pa-hoy-hoy) and a'a (ah ah). Pahoehoe lava comes out smooth and dense and can form large areas that resemble flat parking lots or smooth bumps. A'a, on the other hand, forms individual rocks anywhere from a few inches to many feet in size. It is forbidden to take any piece of land/rock from the islands. Stories tell of bad things happening to people who have taken without asking permission. I had received permission from a Kahuna to leave the islands with three rocks.

TSUNAMI HITS

"Life is too vast an ocean to be cast adrift on the atoll of bitterness and regret"
Paul Williams 2009

Hibernation

It was a cold winter day when I arrived in London to a strange mixture of feelings. I felt extremely vulnerable and it was so noisy and the smell was awful as I emerged from the airport terminal building. I had followed my heart and in doing that, I had purged myself of so much emotional, mental, physical and spiritual baggage in following a path towards my soul purpose. I was slightly anxious as to how my parents would receive me and I them, as I knew I felt different. I needn't have worried. It was so good to see them and they both threw their arms around me.

Coming back to where I was born I felt lost. This seemed such a strange land and everything was a shade of grey, seemingly without feeling. I missed the warm tropical weather and smiling faces, beautiful smells and bright colours. This felt like a prison. What was I going to do? I had to find a job, but couldn't bear the thought of working in this country again at this moment in time as it was just too different in the extreme from the environment I had been living in. I had changed and simply couldn't see myself integrating into this inhospitable society. Well that's how it felt.

I stayed with Mum and Dad and I did my best to not intrude. I knew I had changed and I guessed this was being sensed by them at some level. Dad became controlling and wanted to know what I was doing. It seemed like he wanted to put me in a box and I guess he didn't understand why I had given everything up to go to Hawaii, and in his eyes, only to come back with nothing. Little did he know that this had been a most important time in my life and a turning point in my choice to live the life that I wanted. He didn't like me using the computer, even though I was looking for work, so I resorted to going to an internet café in the end to save the tension in the house. I had to get out, not because I didn't love them, but because it wasn't a healthy space for me to be in and I was the cause of the unrest.

I was offered an interview in London in the first week in January, not too long to wait. In the interim, I had a bad cold over Christmas. It was a miserable time. I couldn't seem to relate to my parents at all anymore. So, after the interview I arranged to visit my sister in Ireland to see how her new life was panning out and then to go to see my friend in Spain.

I had a good feeling about the job interview. I had simply expressed who I was and what sort of environment I was looking to work in. I would wait for the results of the interview in Spain, where I felt welcomed. After a week, the call came to say I had been offered a job as a spa manager in the Maldives. It was a dream come true. I had expressed my wish to be in a natural environment by the ocean in a warm country. Through my work experiences I had the ability to adapt to most things and they had a management position which I could easily slip into. Although more stressful than practising therapy, I saw it as an opportunity to embrace a new life. A month later I was getting ready to start a new adventure in Asia.

Boundaries

So it was, I said yet another goodbye to my parents and friends. I left the UK on the first stage to visit the head office in Thailand. Bangkok, was an eclectic mix of hustle and bustle. It was humid, noisy, busy and smelly. How on earth could people live like this I thought to myself? Yet it held a kind of magic and charm, a little like my trip to India years before. It was great to meet the team of people that would be my support at the head office whilst I was out in the field and to gain an insight and introduction to the company and its philosophy which was to prepare me for what was to come.

Five days later I was on another plane to Male, the capital city of the Maldives. I arrived at night and after an arduous wait going through the immigration protocol I emerged to a warm smile from a lovely Maldivian man in a white linen uniform. I wasn't alone. Another couple joined me. They had just arrived on another flight and were on honeymoon and ready to start their holiday on the island that I was to call my home for the next year.

We climbed into a speed boat and were promptly invited to remove our shoes. The island had a 'no shoes,' 'no news' policy. I liked the sound of that! It was incredible how the pilot of the boat navigated the water in pitch black. Twenty minutes later after an exhilarating ride under the stars of the night sky we arrived at the wooden jetty to disembark. I was met by the existing spa manager and shown to my room.

Part of the deal working as an expatriate manager from overseas was that you lived in single accommodation and I knew that I would need my own space. It was also an essential part of the protocol to be respected and create appropriate boundaries. You needed to show a certain rank, rather like being in the Army again, and with that came privileges whether I liked it or not. They had said I would have my own house, a Bubble they called them. The room I was shown to was nothing like what had been described to me. The spa manager told me it was temporary as they didn't have a spare bubble for me at the moment, but would move me into one as soon as possible.

My room was tiny. It had a single bed, an old wooden wardrobe and a table. The toilet and shower was just a tiled open room with no shelving, mirror or cabinets, just plain and simple. There was a gap at the top of the partition and I could hear snoring from the next room. It was like a prison room. In any other circumstance this wouldn't have worried me and I would have just got on with it, but this was going to be my home for at least the next year and how could I retain my integrity and uphold a status when I had no privacy.

Too tired to comment, I unpacked and fell into bed. The next day, I woke up and, for the first time, saw where I had landed in all its glory. I looked out over the wall to a blue ocean. The sun was shining brightly and the sea was gently lapping onto the pure white sandy beach. The colour of the water merged into a beautiful turquoise which continued for about one hundred and fifty metres getting darker in colour until the edge of the reef where it changed into a deep dark blue. Gentle waves broke over the reef giving a sense of protection from the vastness of the ocean. In the distance a dot of land, another island in paradise, showed we weren't completely alone in this vast expanse.

The island was just four hundred metres long and one hundred metres wide and only a metre above sea level. It was a mere speckle of a jewel in this huge ocean. There were three long wooden jetties, spreading like tentacles from the island. All the guest villas were of wooden structures, with Cajun roofs, built over the reef bed. Looking out towards the east of the island was the spa, again built over the water. All treatment rooms had glass bottom panels where any amount of tropical fish would go about their daily business as guests relaxed looking down mesmerised during their massage. Each treatment room had its own uninterrupted view of the reef surf in the distance.

On the west of the island was the main bar and lunchtime restaurant, another wooden structure built over the water, where reef sharks would prowl, waiting for any morsel of food that found its way into the water.

For guests it really was paradise on earth, even the colours were healing and soothing. The warm Indian Ocean and shallow reef was truly a blessing and a diver's paradise. The reef bed had been damaged by the El Nino effect however, the brightly coloured fish made up for anything lacking in the coral. During my time there, I managed to enjoy a couple of dives where the wall of the reef teemed with angelic, weird and wonderful looking fish. The sun was intensely strong during the day and around sunset the mosquitoes would come out in force attacking any juicy white skin around.

There were so many faces. Over two hundred and sixty host staff lived on this tiny island. The level of service was high. There were six members of staff to one villa and people paid a lot of money to come here. The host living area was intense. There were four blocks of two story rooms like mine and you had to walk through the accommodation area to get through to the back of house operations of the host staff quarter.

Self sufficient in almost every way, we drank sea water that had been desalinated which left you with a craving for anything sweet. Power was produced on the island as was sewage treatment. There was a stark looking canteen, a soccer field, made of sand of course, a mosque and a round thatched roofed bar, for social entertainment in the evenings. Concluding our support was the human resources training department, laundry and a tailor. There was everything that was required to support a community of people. We didn't wear shoes in the guest area, but you really wanted to in the host area. The guys had a habit of spitting their guts up into the sand and the noise of this annoyed me intensely. It's a normal practise in this part of the world, but I never got used to it!

I found myself having to adapt radically and quickly, I would not have survived a single month otherwise. It was a completely different world. There were no boundaries, being difficult to have when you live on top of each other, and I really struggled in the beginning. I was located on the top floor in what was apparently one of the nicer rooms. At least I had a room to myself, most shared. They didn't mind this as many lived in one room houses at home and they were used to sharing space with siblings. Actually, when some were given the opportunity to have a single room they chose not too, preferring to share a room with another.

However, for me it was essential for my own boundaries. I'd been born into a different world, where that kind of closeness and living on top of each other was alien. In my world, strong houses were built with separate compartments to enable our individuality to flourish in its own space, rightly or wrongly. The western mentality was just different.

I was grateful to experience living in the host area, although it didn't seem like it at the time, as it gave me insight into the mentality of the people that I was going to be working with. The first morning, I was collected and taken to breakfast. When I walked into the canteen everyone stared. I was so out of place. The spa Manager, an English teacher, and myself were the only white females working on the island. The majority were men from Maldives, Sri Lanka and India. Of a total workforce of two hundred and sixty, approximately eighteen were women. It was geared up to cater for the male population for sure!

Breakfast was an experience. There was curry, curry, some more curry, chapattis and rice. Thankfully I saw a bowl full of Rice Crispies, something familiar, which I had with UHT milk and a cup of Liptons tea. I couldn't bear the thought of eating curry first thing in the morning, not right now, there were too many other strange things to get used to! The canteen was an austere environment, noisy and smelly and you felt like you wanted to wash everything again. That feeling didn't last. I soon got into the swing of things and those stuck up prejudices that I had soon broke down and I found myself embracing the whole thing. After a couple of weeks, I would sit with the guys and communicate with them through physical gestures, eye contact and very broken English. They only really wanted to know if I was married and had children and where I came from, that was our main topic of conversation. I would ask after their families and children, all of whom were miles away. We shared a commonality in being away from friends and family and this was our bond.

My first day in the spa was great. I met the team, happy smiling faces all of them. There were eight different nationalities, mainly women which gave such a different feel to the island gang. Because of our location we were largely left alone, only interacting with the rest of the hosts during mealtimes and after work. I had more interaction with the management team, through meetings and battling to get things done. The spa manager was in the last month of her contract so at least I had some time to adjust whilst she was still here. She was South African and I was very glad of her company. I began to realise the enormity of what I had taken on. When she left, I felt like I was really on my own. There was just the English teacher whom I could have a woman to woman chat with, even then she had been there so long and had a Maldivian boyfriend so our out of hours time was limited.

It was tricky gaining confidence from the guys, especially for me as a single white female manager. The hierarchy was strong and things needed to get done. I had to spend time getting to know them, before they would give me anything. You couldn't shout, certainly not in the beginning, they could make your life hell if they wanted. It was a case of 'slowly, slowly catchy monkey' to gain respect. It was very frustrating when the work ethic in the UK already has a base level of procedures and the simplest things get done. Here you had to chase every moment and every day for the same smallest thing and in most cases there was no sense of urgency. Everyone looked busy, but wasn't really. It was exhausting.

I struggled with my accommodation and not having any privacy or my own space. The noise disturbed me as they would all go to bed so late and had no respect for others. It didn't matter to them, they were used to this. I was getting used to the responsibility of my position and had no thinking time. I was working long hours, six days a week and my day off was for sleeping and housekeeping. I was promised my bubble would be ready soon. They were dragging their feet and I eventually got so angry that I spoke with the general manager and told him this wasn't the deal I signed up for. It was sorted within a week.

The general manager was an affable Aussie, strong, experienced and knew what he was doing. We got on great, although I didn't see much of him occasionally we would have lunch together. He was very interested in my ideas and would play devils advocate where necessary, giving me great support. I was largely left alone to run the spa. My own bosses were based in Thailand and once a week we would have a conference call via Skype to report on business and any other challenges. This took some time to get used to as communication was difficult at the best of times. Telephone calls were extremely expensive and getting a suitable time to call was even more of a challenge. However, for me it was great to have that level of freedom, the ability to make my own decisions in the moment, knowing you were trusted.

On the other hand I lacked emotional support, someone to share frustrations and experience with from my perspective.

Sanctuary

At last I moved into my bubble. Phew, what a relief! There was a side gateway which led into a small sandy garden, surrounded at the back by shrubbery and trees. Beyond that was the pathway to the spa, the beach and ocean. To the sides I was enclosed by white washed walls. The bubble itself was a round structure with a thatched roof. It was open plan inside with a small lounge and day bed area, opening on to the bedroom and outside through a door was the bathroom. The sink and bath were under the roof, but my favourite bit was the shower, which was on the enclosing wall completely open under the sun and the stars at night. I loved having a shower in the morning under the gentle sunrise and equally at night under the bright stars, particularly at full moon.

I made it my home. At last I had some privacy. I kept the blinds shut as you never knew who would pop their head around and come into the garden and as the sun was so strong it was a relief from the intensity of daylight. It was my sanctuary. At first the team wanted to come round so I had to say very clearly that this was my space and I needed this to think. That was the problem you see, I had no contemplation time, which wasn't good as I needed to think strategically for the business.

It took me a long time to get them to understand that. I certainly didn't have any peace at work, my office was shared and nothing was my own and there was an acute lack of operational space. This was something I came to realise would happen at the design stage on most of the projects I have worked on since then. Spas would be built from a visual perspective with very little thought to the operation! I had to learn to go with the flow at work. When I did find time to be alone in the office and close the door, all hell would break out and they would think I wasn't supporting them. It was like managing a group of kindergarten children!

In essence, we were all in the same boat, away from our families, thrown together on a tiny island all from different cultures and beliefs. The spa was a loving place. There would be the odd tantrum from therapists who would fall out over the simplest tiny thing, but it wouldn't last long. We shared a lot and I became their mother and would give advice on anything and everything. Many times I was the mediator, but they gave me so much love back and I will never forget that.

As a female manager, I had to be extremely conscious of my actions and words. Under no circumstances could I relax and have normal friendly banter with the locals. I could smile and laugh and joke, but not like I would in the West. It was dangerous to get too close to anyone of them. Gossip was rife and could potentially destroy you. I saw it happen to our general manager when he got too close to one of the girls. The guys ganged up on him and took revenge by getting him the sack. The English teacher who was involved with one of the local guys found her life wasn't her own anymore as possessiveness, control and jealousy took over.

As new therapists arrived, I counselled them about not getting too close, particularly in the beginning, when they were vulnerable and told them to bide their time as it would save them a lot of pain in the long run. If you tried to get out of a relationship or friendship, a vendetta would evolve out of all proportion. That's when I became very glad of my need to be insular. It was survival, made easy because of my position. Island life was intense and many expats simply couldn't cope.

At first, I really struggled in myself as it felt like mental and emotional torture here. I disliked the lack of respect for space and privacy and I desperately tried to hold on to a sense of 'me.' I had to do things I really didn't like doing, because I was tired. Every month we would have a host party. It was a big deal and those with families living on the main capital of Male were invited to join the melee. Every month we would put on a show. There would be live music and awards and sometimes we did a superstar competition and enjoyed a fantastic buffet BBQ themed spread.

As part of the executive committee we, the management team, would have to stand on the stage like lemons and do a little speech on something and then present the prizes. I loved that bit! It was the whole showmanship that I struggled with. My shyness would bubble up to the surface as it seemed like eyes bore straight through me. I wanted to hide! Anyway, I would simply take a deep breath and go with the flow.

Part of the problem was that I had very little energy for extracurricular activities as I was always extremely tired. Working six days a week and long hours meant I would fall into bed at night, grateful for my sleep, so these events were more of a drain and I would leave as soon as the awards were over. It sounds really selfish, but I had nothing left to give. Days off were spent trying to relax and switch off my mind. That was pretty challenging as I was always thinking about work. Occasionally I would catch the dhoni into Male – a one hour roller coaster ride by boat. It was brave as I knew sea sickness was a possibility, but I wanted to experience the capital city, and what an experience. I thought I stuck out like a sore thumb on the island, but our guys were pussy cats compared to city life!

Men would stare and their eyes were cold, unforgiving and mistrustful. As a Muslim country, of course you would cover up, you wouldn't dream of not doing so, but it didn't matter. Walking through the shopping area was hassle. Going into shops was not a pleasant experience as you would be shadowed around the shop and it felt like you were a criminal. The supermarkets were fine as they were much more open and modern.

I would close down completely anytime I went there. I found a western style coffee shop where I would indulge in a latte and wait for the dhoni to return. It was a little piece of my old culture! Needless to say I didn't venture into town much.

After about four months, I was settled into a routine but by this time I was really exhausted as island life took its toll. The team was fragile emotionally. I found that if I withdrew and tried to work in my office on strategic ideas for the business, the wheels would fall of and discord would reign. The balance was to be there with the team, cajoling, checking and supporting most of the time and then work on reports and other admin when I got home.

I was overdue some rest and recuperation time. It was recommended you take a break after three months. My friend from the UK wanted to visit so we compromised. She would come and stay for a week on the island then together we would fly to Goa for a week. I was worried about leaving the team, but so desperately needed some time away. I left my assistant manager in charge.

Goa was lovely. Funnily enough, we arrived out of season, so the hotel was full of conference delegates, all male, staring at us white females. I couldn't get away from it! Oh well, I was determined to enjoy some relaxation. Our room wasn't good and we complained. It didn't match the description and it turned out they had down graded us! It was put right after a complaint to the manager and we ended up in a very good room indeed.

A week was too short. I was still on tenterhooks and felt at breaking point. I'd had enough and wanted to give it all up but I had another seven months to go before the end of my contract. Thank goodness for my friend. She helped me remember where I had come from. So, I said goodbye to her at the airport and as the speedboat bought me closer back to the island, I began to sense something was up.

True to my feeling, there was indeed uneasiness in the air. The team wouldn't look at me. I sensed a real discord. It didn't take long to discover that my assistant manager had been gossiping and manipulating the truth. I knew she was ambitious, but I was still surprised that she would do this and I felt hurt.

Thankfully, one by one my team came to me with their stories. We began to smile and joke again and they would pile into my office and create merry hell, but I knew I wouldn't have it anyway other way. The feeling when I returned was not pleasant at all. I believe if I hadn't had such a good relationship with each one of them I would have gone the same way as others before and my life would have been made impossible. Gossip kills that's for sure, particularly in a close knit community. The main issue with my deputy was that she started to be very dictatorial and would shout and bully the team. She would say that is how I should be managing the spa. It made me think about my own style of management.

Then I would see the whole picture and realise that we had a harmonious team and the standards were high even though it took me three months to get a simple system like the room set up right! In military style, without the shouting, every morning I would take each individual into their treatment room and go through it like a fine toothcomb. They now knew the set up exactly to standard. It took a lot of initial effort on my part but I wouldn't have it any other way.

In the mornings at 11am we would have thirty minutes together as a team and sit in the Yoga Champa on the beach. Sometimes I would take them into a guided meditation and relaxation, sometimes a Tai Chi session with one of our therapists. Initially there was a lot of giggling, but I was determined to set the scene for us all to have this sacred space together as a support for each other. Occasionally, we would miss a session for one reason or another and we all missed it when it happened. My management style was about cooperation not destruction or fear.

We had a regular evening together once a month, just the spa team. We would sometimes go into Male for a meal, leaving on the late dhoni after closing, sometimes we'd hire a speed boat and dance the night away at Club Med an island about twenty minutes away. They were good times and an opportunity for me to let my hair down far away from prying eyes. My team was multinational and worldlier. We did laugh and dance a lot.

Eventually, we were joined by my other hosts who we, as a team, worked more closely with. It opened up and strengthened the connection with the resort hosts. Slowly my social life improved and I started to enjoy going off island with the general manager, managers and the dive team for the odd trip to the airport hotels to enjoy meeting other expats. The dive team were a franchise and, in a way, independent from the company I worked for, but I spent more time with them than anyone else. But island life is incredibly intense; every little thing is really a big thing.

South American flavour

One day the dive manager introduced me to Carlos his new dive master. What a hunk! He was from Columbia, fit, sexy, and he knew it, with a wonderful accent. He was like something out of a movie. I wondered why he would come to such a remote place.

Anyhow, all the girls were tittering away and the dive centre became a babe magnet. The social scene on the island had been gathering pace and our host bar became the hub for birthday parties, in fact, for any excuse for a celebration. The spa team were always present at these events. Of course, it helped that we were mostly female. There were only three males in our team! The girls were the belles of the ball. The island seemed to become less intense, or so it seemed. My view point probably changed because I was more relaxed and accepting of island life, knowing I didn't have long left of my contract. We enjoyed a great rapport in the spa team, no real problems there, and business was doing very well too.

Carlos was the new idol. He had bought some South American music and once a week in our sand pit of a bar the music would play and we learned how to salsa and merengue. Carlos he knew his stuff! He never got involved publicly with anyone, I am not sure what he did behind closed doors but I didn't hear any gossip. He became part of our social group. I got on well with Carlos. I was about four years older than him and the young girls would flirt around him like bees around a honeypot, it was very amusing.

One evening he came with us to the airport hotel to celebrate the general manager's birthday. Later in the evening I was with Carlos talking with some other people and the general manager came up to us and slapped us both on the back and blatantly said in a loud voice, "When the hell are you two going to get it together then!?" Carlos and I just looked at each other and laughed. Some sort of magic started to happen and we both went all coy and shy! Obviously there was truth in what he had said.

Someone else then said to me that Carlos couldn't take his eyes off me. I didn't believe them, thinking this was a conspiracy. I was at this time very closed. Anyway, I thought there is no way that I could get involved with anyone on the island. I would be doomed!

We sat next to each other on the boat ride back to the island. There was that spark of electricity between us. It would be lovely to have a hug and be close to someone and my mind started to work overtime. We walked slowly down the jetty and as everyone peeled off to go back home, we ended up walking in the same direction.

As we came near to my pad, he said, "Can I come in?"

"Yes," I said.

Oh my God, what am I doing? Jane no, not again! Oh but wouldn't it be so good. It doesn't have to be serious. A battle was raging in my mind. Then I decided. "Jane you only live once. He is single. You are single. There is nothing wrong with this." Decision made. He stayed the night. I was in heaven. He was the most considerate lover I had ever experienced. We agreed that this was just what it was and between us only. He left in the early hours of the morning before sunrise. That was a huge relief to me. I didn't want anyone to know as my life would be hell if anyone found out.

In between the night times and when I was alone, I felt on the edge, like I was holding on for dear life. I was desperately lonely, probably the loneliest I have ever felt in my life. The smallness of the island and the vastness of the universe that you could see at night added to that feeling. Carlos was an interlude, a commercial break. The reality was I had no-one to have a real good chat to, because of the small community it was impossible to have any privacy. Communications were poor and calls extremely expensive. Skype was hit and miss and my friends were far away not just in distance but in time difference too. I spoke to my parents once in a while and they always knew if I wasn't happy. I tried to keep my conversations light hearted with them, hiding the reality of how I was really feeling. I spoke with my friend in Spain. I remember once I was able to tell her how I felt and it made me realise how isolated I really was. I missed my friends and family. It doesn't matter how many people there are around you, it's what's going on inside that counts.

Our guests were normally reasonable and affluent people. There were a few difficult characters to deal with, who were on some sort of personal ego trip, which added to the pressure. It could be an emotional ride. I had very little connection with the land or the people. Although I adored my team, they were so sensitive and would pick up straight away if I was under the weather or feeling particularly stressed so I really had to put on a 'show' as otherwise they would sense something was wrong and it would affect everyone. The whole situation was raw and fragile. Anything could tip the balance either way. It was a huge responsibility trying to hold the space and I was suffering inside and I guess still grieving for the loss of my baby and the huge experience I had in Hawaii.

I had a couple of months left of my contract and there was no way I wanted to stay, paradise or not. It was an extreme polarity. Guests would often say to me how lucky I was. I would say to them, yes, I walk to work on white sand everyday and have this permanent view of the beautiful blue ocean, yet I still have the stress and pressure of being away from my friends and family and the pressures of running a business, having to hold myself together and be strong emotionally for everyone and all with very little support. There is always a flip side.

For the past two months we had had a construction team working on a new huge exclusive villa out in the lagoon. The project manager was American and he stayed on the island with us. John's workforce stayed on a nearby local island. We became friends, another breath of normality, a fellow partner in crime. We would only get together at lunch and perhaps if I went to the bar in the evening. It was someone familiar to chat to. It helped. Carlos was my secret and we would not get together again until Christmas time. I was so grateful for that interaction. I felt like a human being again, a female and really it had done me the world of good.

Christmas was looming yet it didn't feel christmassy at all. It was blazing hot, the resort was about seventy percent full and a different kind of guest arrived for the Christmas week. We decorated the spa with palm tree leaves around the wooden pillars and the gardeners made beautiful palm displays with the coconut pods and buds. It was all very natural, low key and in tune with our environment. Although we were in a Muslim country, as a resort we catered for and celebrated all religious and important dates in the diary. The majority of our guests for the festive season were from the West.

Fighting for life

On Christmas Eve a small group of us, including John and Carlos, went to the airport Hotel to escape. We weren't required for work and it was a great opportunity to mingle with other expats celebrating Christmas. That night Carlos stayed again. He left early Christmas day morning.

The guests were happy and enjoying Christmas day in the sunshine. We shut the spa at lunchtime and ordered some takeaway pizza from Male which was a boat trip away. One of our team went off to collect the pizzas. It would take about an hour. In the meantime, we decorated the upstairs relaxation area, put all our presents on the table and waited for our pizzas to arrive. We were all very excited. Even the non Christians joined in. It was yet another beautiful day and the pizzas arrived and we sat on the floor and shared food, stories and presents. It was a very special time. We took the rest of the day off.

Christmas day night, we gathered in the sand pit bar for a few drinks and then I took the opportunity of having an early night. Around seven thirty in the morning on Boxing day I felt the ground shake. I often felt the atoll shake, but this one was a little stronger than normal.

Then I had to rush to the toilet as I had diarrhoea, very strange as I normally have a cast iron stomach. The shaking continued for a while, then settled down. I wanted to enjoy a day on the beach. I didn't very often do this as normally I just wanted to hide away in my room and rest. But it was such a glorious day and it was Boxing day.

I plastered my body with suntan lotion as the sun was extreme here, put my costume on and grabbed my towel and a book and walked out down the path towards the ocean. It was a strange sight. The beach had all but disappeared. This was abnormal. When we had a full moon the tide was always higher but what struck me was the choppy water. It was very unusual to see the reef water choppy. The sun was brilliant, not a cloud in the sky. I looked over to the spa and saw my girls running across the jetty; at the same time I noticed the water level had risen so much it was the same level as the spa and rising.

I started to run towards the spa, concerned for the girls. I didn't get there, as what I can only describe as a huge volume of water gushed onto the island. It just kept coming. I got swept along back down the path, past my home. I had no control and was not able to fight against the flow. I let go and allowed the water to take me. As I was carried swiftly across to the other side of the island, I saw this poor guy in a buggy and, as I passed, I shouted for him to get out. I could see he was in shock and didn't know what to do. We glanced at each other in disbelief, as I flowed past. I lost sight of him and I noticed one of my shoes bobbing along in the water. I grabbed it and held on to it. Everything was in slow motion. When I looked towards the direction I was going, I saw the sea level rise in front of me and suddenly the land disappeared completely. I was still over the island, but in water. A surreal thought came into my mind. What if the earth doesn't come back? I felt very grateful for being a strong fearless swimmer in that moment.

The flow slowed and I managed to find my feet on something and slowly waded towards the restaurant building which was on slightly higher ground. As I turned the corner, most of the guests who had been enjoying a late breakfast were now wet up to their waists in water and in shock.

My mind kicked into action as I began to worry about the spa. Who was in treatment rooms? Did everyone get out? The flow had eased and I waded back through the water, checking on people as I went. They were all in shock. Thankfully, I found my team all together. A couple of them had climbed up the palm trees in fear as they couldn't swim. Everyone was safe. We waded towards the dive centre which was the highest place and was a two story building. Faces were grey, all the smiles had disappeared completely.

Crisis management

All the managers met with the general manager and we made a plan to do a headcount of both hosts and guests. John and I worked together in accounting for the guests. I had already been able to account for my own team and they were safe and gathered in one place. I asked my team to look after any of the families and assist where possible if they could.

The staff of the resort, particularly the butlers and guest relations were brilliant. They arranged to rescue guests who were trapped in their villas. The jetties had been ripped up by the force of the water. Almost every villa had been damaged, some so severely that there was hardly anything left. After a fraught couple of hours we had accounted for everyone. Everyone was safe with only a few minor cuts and scraps. There was incredible damage to the infrastructure for almost everywhere had been destroyed or severely damaged except the dive centre and the spa. By this time we had got word of what had happened elsewhere. Male had been hit, but no major damage, the airport had been swamped, but not damaged and the water had receded.

Our office manager in Male was busy organising to get our guests off our island, which was now a very unsafe place to be. Over the next six hours guests had a choice, they could go to another resort and continue their holiday as not all resorts had been hit, or they could get to the airport and wait for a flight home. We had no way to look after them. Most decided to go home with the rest going on to another resort.

It's amazing how people react in times of crisis and when their survival is threatened. Some go into a cocoon and need holding; others become warriors and protectors and hide all emotion. Underneath all of this there was a constant fear of this happening again, as we were now aware of what had happened, although not to what extent elsewhere. Tsunami became the big word. We provided life jackets to the hosts and got all those on the ground floor to move in with those on the top floor of the accommodation blocks that weren't damaged. We all worked tirelessly to start the long process of cleaning up the enormous amount of debris and to making areas safe again for sleeping as we only had this tiny slip of land to be on.

During this time, I went into an upstairs office and, in a blur, called Mum and Dad. I couldn't bear the thought of them seeing this on the television and then worrying. I knew by calling I would wake them, but

I had to do it. The phone rang. I let it ring knowing they may not hear it. Dad answered in a sleepy voice.

I said, "Dad it's me, sorry it's early and I woke you but something has happened and I don't want you to worry. There's been some sort of disaster. We are okay here, damaged buildings but everyone is fine. You may see this on the television, but don't worry as I am fine. I'm not sure how long the telephone lines will be open, so I wanted to phone you while I could".

He said, "Okay Janey, thanks for calling." The line went dead. I had got in just in time. I didn't get to speak to them again for a good few days.

I remember being on a mission to walk the island. I wanted to know where everyone was, who was looking after whom. It was like marking a territory again, wanting to know the boundaries. As we gradually said goodbye to the guests and focussed on being safe for the night ahead, I began to feel really unwell. It was like a wave of flu like symptoms building up in my body. I felt awful but I kept going and didn't stop until that night.

My home had been devastated. It was like a tornado of water had literally lifted and swirled and dumped the contents of my home. The huge heavy furniture had been picked up and left in disarray, turned upside down. The entrance door was blocked with the wardrobe and I got help to try and move this out of the way so I could at least get in to salvage anything left. Ironically, I had packed a suitcase ready for a holiday that I was due to have a week later. The suitcase was sodden with dirty, smelling muddy water. All my clothes, jewellery, computer, books, everything had been under water. Items that were loose were lost to the depths of the Indian ocean. Two of those items were my lovely peridot necklace from Hawaii and one of the stones. I never found my other shoe.

Luckily, I managed to salvage a credit card, a water logged passport and two water logged books and one of my two journals, damaged but salvageable. The other journal of my journey so far in the Maldives was gone. The journal that survived was my record of the months I had spent in Hawaii the previous year. I was still in my costume and had a sarong wrapped around me that had now dried. I was hoping to get some clothes on, but there was nothing left that could be salvaged.

Strangely, I had this urge to get into the ocean, bizarre I know. So I followed that notion. It was a sorry sight as I walked the same way I had gone earlier that day. The tide was very low, the lowest that I had ever seen. Many dead fish were washed up on the shore and brightly coloured corals littered the beach. I walked straight into the ocean, submerged myself and walked out again. It felt like I needed to make friends with the ocean again.

I continued to get worse, headache, achy joints and a streaming cold. It was so sudden. There were three of us who had lost everything we owned and that night we had nowhere to sleep, nowhere safe to run to, so the three of us found some sun loungers in the bar, which had not been damaged. However, the bar was over the water. It was a very strange night, fearful of another wave, all we could hear was the water lapping underneath us. We all waited for any change in the noise denoting a rise in the level. It was a very tense night.

We made a pact, the three of us, that if a wave came again we'd hold on to each other and go together! Night drew in and the mosquitoes came out in vengeance. They don't ever give in! Chris, one of the chefs, and I couldn't sleep. The slightest difference in wave noise and we'd be right awake so we decided to tour the island. It was pitch black and rather a stupid thing to do! We got hold of a torch and ended up in the bar area where a few people had salvaged a bottle of whisky or two and were drowning their sorrows. It looked a right mess. I didn't fancy anything, suffering as I was with a heavy cold or flu, so we circumnavigated the island. The moon was shining brightly. Looking up at the night sky, you would never have known the devastation that had hit the region that day. Now it was calm and serene, the stars shining brightly as if nothing had happened.

The next day, the focus was on the hosts. As part of the management team we had to reintroduce structure and routine as the framework had been broken down. Working parties were set up for each area of the resort. I had no problem with my team as they couldn't wait to get into their beloved spa and start cleaning up. Structurally it had held up quite well, but there was a lot of internal damage.

We took regular breaks and chatted and supported each other as best we could. I was feeling really ill. The guest kitchen and restaurant area thankfully were fairly intact which meant, as we didn't have any guests, we could use their supplies and a mock up kitchen area was put together in our host area. Our own kitchen and staff area had been hit quite badly. The guys did an incredible job of feeding us. It is absolutely inspiring how people come together in times like these.

I was constantly asked by my team about the future. When could they go home? Would they still have a job and if so, how long before they could come back? There was no doubt in their mind that they wanted to come back here. Fearful about supporting their families back home, they needed an income.

The damage to the resort was severe. John, as project manager, had an immense task of reconstructing the whole resort. Within ten days he had rallied up workers from the disaster area. It meant work and food on the table for families. They put up a camp site, on what we named Sahara beach, for the three hundred workers due on site. A week earlier Sahara beach had been the romantic setting for the weekly cocktail party for the guests, now it was full of tents, men and tools. It was a mammoth task.

Meanwhile, we set up two daily briefings to keep up morale and to bond everyone together. Mornings were clean up time and we would gather up debris from around the island, then go on to our own areas to continue cleaning up. Afternoon was accommodation clean up and a bit of socialising time.

I was still feeling incredibly ill. A colleague from my team Rachel, who was a South African lady a couple of years younger than me, had only been with us for a month so this was a real baptism of fire for her. She had changed her whole life around from being in corporate business world into retraining and becoming a therapist. I don't know what I would have done without her. Luckily her room was on the top floor of the accommodation block and intact. I had nowhere to sleep during this time, so she opened up her room to me and I shared that space for the remainder of our time there. The girls gave me t-shirts and shorts to wear and a pair of flip flops, so at least I could be decent!

I was under pressure to keep the girls on the island. It was good for morale the guys said. I had different ideas. To me, it wasn't safe. We were a small team of females in a growing team of men and normality had gone out of the window.

All they wanted to do was to get home to their families and make sure they were safe. I asked the team what they needed to get home in terms of money or tickets etc. To this day I am amazed at the integral way they responded. They gave me a list of exactly what they needed, to the penny. Some didn't want anything as they had family in the country; others needed a small amount of spending money to get them home.

Most of us expats already had return tickets. To get a visa and work in the country you had to come in with a return ticket. We had something called a social fund which had been built up from the service charge that was added on to the guest bill. It was like a guaranteed tip. As all of our salaries were very low, we used this for our nights out and presents or to buy fridges and TV's for the rooms, which, at that time, were not supplied by the company. There was a good amount left and I had to use this money to get them home.

I didn't have any contact from my bosses in Bangkok. The spa was in a separate division to the resort and had different staffing structure and reporting lines. The offices based in Bangkok had closed down for the holiday time. It reopened on the 3rd of January. I didn't receive a call from any one of my immediate bosses to see how we were. This left a bitter taste in my mouth. The owners of the resort company were on their way to the region. They arrived in amongst the debris and spent time with us and I think we were all very grateful that they made the effort as it had a huge impact on the whole team.

No one from our team took advantage of this situation. Over the course of the next week, our numbers slowly diminished as I said goodbye to them for the last time. There were some very sad moments. I couldn't guarantee them anything except that I would do my best to get them a placement elsewhere in the company. It would be nearly a year before the resort would open again.

Finally, the time came for me to leave as well. Rachel and I were the last ones to leave from the Spa team. I left my colleagues with some very unhappy faces that day. It was awful. I left with my passport, a damaged suitcase with hardly anything in it, a borrowed pair of shorts, t-shirt and flip flops. Off I went to Dubai where I bought some clothes and trainers to wear home. The flight was packed back to London.

When we landed, I shall never forget the overwhelming feeling of care from the British people and the announcement on board asking anyone coming from the disaster area to make themselves known to the police who were coming aboard as people needed to be accounted for. This lovely man came up to me and said, "Are you okay? "

I blubbered through tears and said, "Yes."

He said, "We have a team of counsellors here to help you. Do you have someone to meet you?"

I said "I am okay, my parents are coming to greet me."

The overwhelming sense of support that followed was humbling. I arrived again in the cold winter time. Mum and Dad were again very glad to see me, but there was a change. They couldn't do enough for me. I really felt cared for. It was such a contrast to a year or so earlier, when I came back from Hawaii. "How can we help you, what can we do?" They would turn off the news, seeing that it upset me and nothing was too difficult for them. They watched me like a hawk. In reality, I was still in shock.

I was still the manager of the spa with my contract just about finished and I still had responsibilities to find the team a place to go. We had just opened a big spa in Dubai and luckily it was their busy season so most of my therapists were offered a position there. Only a couple decided to take time out and regroup and wait for our island to reopen. Sadly, I never saw any of them again.

BABBLING BROOKS

> "Experience life in all possible ways — good-bad, bitter-sweet, dark-light, summer-winter. Experience all the dualities. Don't be afraid of experience, because the more experience you have, the more mature you become."
> Osho

Aftermath

Waves of anger, sadness and despair filled me like the Tsumani itself. It had been a week since returning from the tsunami area. I hadn't felt anything at the time, except numbness and feeling really unwell with my body hurting all over. Now, back in the UK, feelings and emotions started to bubble up to the surface. News bulletins flooded my psyche and I couldn't seem to get away from it. Everywhere people were talking about it. Every newspaper and magazine had images of the complete devastation it had caused and the outpouring of compassion and help from all over the world. It seemed unreal and I felt very lonely.

I felt so sad for those left behind after losing a loved one. I felt for those wandering around still in shock, not knowing what had hit them. I felt guilty, but also grateful, for being alive. A real duality of emotions and feelings. As I checked my emails the week following the disaster, my team would ask me daily if I had received a call from our head office. I had not. It was a blow to them, as they wanted to know that there had been some concern for us all. I also wanted to know that I had support. It bothered my team and now it bothered me. Why hadn't they called? The resort managers had regular contact with our owners and they had come to visit us. Where were my bosses? It was as if we had been abandoned and I knew some of them were not in the region at the time and hadn't been affected directly. They probably thought that I would manage as that was the norm, however, I was managing on the surface but beneath I was distraught and my raw emotions were never far from the surface.

I finally received contact from our head office via email from our managing director's PA. She said that our managing director had been trapped in Borneo and was unable to make contact with the outside world during the disaster as the government there had restricted communications. I felt relieved and a little guilty for feeling angry in the way I did. However, there were others in our support group who could have made contact with us as they were based outside of the area at the time. There was really no excuse. The head office had closed down for the Christmas break, but it was not as if they did not know what had happened. I can only surmise that they thought we were all right.

Gratefully, I received a call from my managing director as soon as he was able to make contact. Of course, I was back in the UK by then, but the call was appreciatively received by me as I could hand over the responsibility for finding my team work as I had promised and could get on with getting myself together.

Once I had offloaded on him, poor guy! I began to feel better. The aches had all but gone and my headaches abated. Inside I felt fearful and jumpy, like my core was shattered. Slowly, I began to take on the enormity of what had happened. I still could not watch or read anything about the disaster. It was too raw.

Mum and Dad showed real concern and could not seem to do enough for me. I remembered that they were like this after the rape incident, even though they didn't know what had happened. I felt genuine caring love. They were glad that I was alive. Dad was incredibly sensitive and continued to turn off the television when the news bulletins came on and they would listen when I talked. It was a loving time of which I shall never forget.

After a couple of weeks, I began to feel the pressure of needing to get back to work. There was no way I wanted to go back to the Maldives, so I discussed options with my company. A new project in Crete had come up, with a position to oversee a new spa project development, train a team and generally be the lynch pin in all aspects of setting up and opening the spa. It was not due to start for another month or so and I needed a proper holiday as I was incredibly exhausted and needed to make sense of my feelings again and discover what this was all about.

I was in a similar space to the one I was in after my experience a year earlier when I had lost my baby. Fragile, vulnerable and like a newborn baby. This time though, the experience had affected many thousands of people from all over the world and I was not alone. What a reflection. Being back with my parents was good, but I needed to be in an environment that was nourishing from an elemental perspective and one that would enable me to feel supported on all levels.

So it was that I booked to take a holiday in Hawaii. It was a familiar sacred place for me to go. I wasn't under pressure to get back to work anytime soon, and I was very grateful for that. Hawaii, being a natural healing space, was the perfect bolthole.

Sacred sanctuary

On the 30th January 2005 I found myself on a flight to Los Angeles. I broke up the journey with an overnight stop, and then woke early to get to the airport for the onward flight to Kahului, Maui. What a mess at the airport. There were so many people and long, long queues to get through security. The legacy of 9/11 still rattled on. I was really glad that I had turned up extra early. As I got on the plane to Maui, I felt quite tearful. It was the thought of going home to Hawaii, rather than the experience I had just been through, I began to relax for the first time in over a year. As we flew near the islands, I realised how far away from myself I had come. I was unfit, stressed, completely exhausted and I had no motivation to do anything. I felt bereft and empty.

I began to realise how lonely, anxious, fearful and sad I had been in the Maldives but now I was beginning to feel connected again, particularly to the beautiful land of the islands. I had planned a healing journey with Nicole, and before that, I used the first week as grounding and nourishment for my body, which was hurting deeply.

My 'journey' with Nicole, was gentle and normal, no heavy stuff. As I was in that newborn baby stage, I was like a blank sheet of paper. It was a blessing to choose how I wanted to create my life from now on. So, we focussed on the positive and the fact that I could create a life that made my heart and soul sing. We went back to basics, discovering what made me feel good. I had let go of so much karma, stuff, baggage, whatever you want to call it. The tsunami was another level of cleansing on a much more global level. There was some residue still to arise as I was still suffering from the after affects of being involved with such a disaster. However, somehow deep inside, I was alright. I felt connected again and no longer alone. Out of the heaviness of grief, lightness emerged.

During the second week, I travelled to Kaua'i for the first time. There I was to meet up with my friend Lucy. It was the first time she had been on such a long haul flight. We had met a few years earlier at a meditation group I used to go to and I felt very closely linked with her. We felt safe together.

Kaua'i is the oldest of the Hawaiian chain of islands and completely different to Maui, rugged, strong, yet with gentleness. The ocean seemed to emanate more power and turbulence here. We had not planned anything and wanted to go with the flow. After a couple of days relaxing and settling in, we decided to take ourselves off on some adventures. I was feeling good and excited about discovering this new land. Little did I know it would end up being an eye opening past life adventure and very resonant with my time in Hawaii before, just over a year ago.

It was a fine sunny morning as we set out from our digs towards Wailua Valley. We drove along and got to the end of the road, looked over the cliff down to a stunning waterfall. Rainbow colours hung in the mist as the force of the water tumbled over the precipice, crashing below into the meandering river. We both looked at each other and thought the same, how fantastic would it be to get down to the bottom!

We could not see anyway down from where we were, so we backtracked and pulled off road, where we noticed what looked like a path leading down into the ravine. It was high up as you could see the tops of the trees from where we stood. We were looking at the top of a forest canopy. Driven by some sort of instinct, we decided to follow the track down the steep cliff face.

The track soon became lost in roots and shrubbery and our path became slippery and dangerous. Any sensible person would probably have turned back! For some unknown reason we kept going down and down, using the strong roots of the trees, which were clinging to the side of the ravine, for support. The trees became our friends and they guided us down to the river below. The treacherous path down was well worth the risk. It was such a beautiful day, not a cloud in the sky. There had been some recent rain and I was fully aware of the dangers of flash floods, but it felt absolutely right that we were there. For the next hour or so, we enjoyed bathing in the cool crystal clear water, laying on the rocks, meditating and embracing the awesome energy of this valley. I allowed my thoughts and feelings to flow. The cool water was nourishing. During one of my meditations I saw a scene play out which somehow put a perspective on the physical and emotional pain that I had suffered when I miscarried fourteen months earlier. Let me explain.

I never thought I would believe in past life experiences, but since I had studied and practised different healing modalities and meditations over the years, I knew unresolved past life issues, karma for want of a better word, had a part to play in our current lives.

All the experiences from before birth, in my mothers' womb, my choice of parents, partners, friends and circumstances have played a part in allowing me to become conscious and choose to release unhealthy patterns and beliefs. I am not a victim of circumstance, although in the beginning it seemed I was. That inner strength and sense of adventure that is unconsciously there inside, drove me towards consciousness and awareness. The pain and suffering I experienced was an opportunity in this lifetime, to finally do something about it. I came to recognise that the power of attachments, in any sense, and on any level can create unhealthy as well as healthy patterns in life. It is all a matter of choice. We are all given opportunities to wake up to a different reality, many of us choose not to and continue to live in the drama that is pain and suffering. We attract that which may need attention or observation, be it people, events or life situations. Every breath we take is valid. Every experience is valid it's simply whether or not we choose to notice and to deal with them. If we chose to work with our experiences we are striving to live a fulfilling life, not only for ourselves but for the good of all those around us.

The real life journeys and all the healing and teachings I have received both physically, mentally, emotionally and spiritually over the years have allowed me to clear my clutter so far. This lifetime has for me been, in so many ways, a baptism of fire and it has allowed me to release the ties that have bound me into making the same painful choices in all of my lives so far. I still have a long way to go!

So, here I am, sun pouring down into the valley, not a cloud in the sky. I closed my eyes and I saw myself living an idyllic life in Hawaii with the feeling of family support, living in an indigenous village in ancient times. The huts were basic, but life was full of love. Fresh food was in abundance. Tropical fruits, vegetables and beautiful flowers were part of everyday life. I was in love and a strong sense of balance and harmony prevailed in our community. I saw that I had long flowing hair with flowers tucked behind my ears. It truly was paradise.

On what seemed like a similar day, bright, warm and clear, in my vision I saw that I was pregnant and very happy. There were a few of us girls together who went down to the river to collect water, singing and chanting as we went, cooling our bodies in the water. Out of the blue, warriors appeared. faces dark with anger and brandishing spears, running through the stream, killing all in their wake. There was such anger and rage in these men, hatred burned in their eyes. A warrior came up to me and stabbed me in the stomach. I screamed in pain and was completely shocked at this attack on my being. It seemed like the first time in my life I had ever experienced anger and such destruction. I screamed, "How dare you, you've killed my baby!" As I fell to the ground, I was already losing my life, but could still see the whole scene. I wanted to hit out and grab this man and scream at him, but no words would ever come out. It was too late to say anything. As my consciousness left my body, I felt my baby was still alive. Then the vision ended. I was shaking with rage and in tears as the memory of fourteen months ago came flooding back. It was as if Adam had stabbed me in the stomach again.

I was a few boulders away from Lucy. I sat with this vision for a while then got myself together and left a flower to drift down the river. We sat in silence and ate our sandwiches. Just as we were finishing our lunch, I had a very strong feeling of fear wash over me.

I said to Lucy, "Look, there's a cloud."

In that moment she also said, "I'm feeling fear. Let's get out of here!"

Urgency helped us both to scramble back up the ravine in record time. Where we got the strength from I have no idea, but both of us were gasping for breath as we reached the top just as the clouds really came into the valley.

We both reflected on our experience later that day. It was very poignant that I saw this past life vision as it made me realise that there have been many past life experiences that have had relevant lessons for me in this lifetime. I was so grateful that Lucy was here with me sharing the energy of the islands and this revelation. It could have been a different outcome had I not had her support. I was still in a very fragile state of fear at my core.

We continued, over the next couple of days, to visit special places of interest and opening up to even more vivid visions and energies. I was really getting a clear out, almost like a spiritual tsunami in itself, the reality of which now seemed like a lifetime ago. Every now and then, I would have a flashback and feelings of fear would consume me, but generally, I felt safe here.

I always dreamed of having a home here on one of the islands, somewhere I could come and stay part of the year but had I had no idea how that could ever come about. One evening we went to a café off the beaten track, where they were serving good home cooked food. We sat in a covered garden area and live musicians were playing. Lucy and I enjoyed a lovely meal and as we were having dessert, a group converged into the tiny remaining space. They were an interesting gaggle of people and we soon got chatting. There was a man, perhaps in his sixties, neatly dressed with a bright white set of teeth. These were the first things you noticed about him.

We chatted for a while and the conversation got a little deeper. It turned out that he owned one of the biggest parks in Kaua'i. He came from a family of missionaries who were first bought into Hawaii following Captain Cook's arrival. It was incredibly interesting and the conversation got onto what we all wanted out of life. Amongst other things, he talked a lot about his painful divorce from his wife, who was taking him to the cleaners. In other words, she wanted his money. Lucy talked about some of her dreams and I mentioned that I was here recovering from being involved in the tsunami and this would be my dream place to live. "Oh, well we have to get you here." he boomed. I laughed. I had heard this before.

Next, he was planning a way to get me here, how he would get me a visa and who knows what after his divorce. My barriers went up, a bit of deja-vu creeping in again. I immediately thought, "There will be another way, right now my integrity is the most important thing." I said, "Thank you, perhaps we can meet up again before we go home," and left it at that. After all it could have been the copious amounts of wine he had been drinking! We did not see him again, but a part of me began to think that my dream was still possible. I was being shown opportunities and possibilities that I never thought would be available again but I would not compromise myself. Another opportunity did arise a couple of years later when I was in a serious relationship with someone.

On the very last day, we visited a Heiau at Lydgate Park. I was with Lucy and a lady who was a friend of someone I knew back in the UK. She lived and worked in Kaua'i. We walked through the park and I began to feel increasingly uncomfortable and upset. I kept walking and came up to the heiau wall, where I fell to my knees and howled for a good half an hour. All the heiau in the islands hold such powerful energy that you cannot help but be moved. I was transfixed, my two friends left me in peace, knowing I was safe. I could not even tell you what it was all about. Maybe it was the shock of my experience back in the Maldives finally surfacing along with the anger and the sorrow of so many lives that had been lost and the grieving families left behind. It felt enormous. When the tears stopped, I went and bathed my feet in the Pacific Ocean for what I thought would be the last time that year. We shared a breakfast and said our goodbyes as we left for the airport for the long flight home.

My heart felt heavy and sad leaving Kaua'i. It had been amazing and well worth the ups and downs. I felt stronger again and rejuvenated, even though it had been an emotional ride. I felt really good internally and externally, cleansed in every sense of the word!

Trapped and facing fear

It was mid February when we arrived back to a cold day in London. Lucy was picked up by her partner and I got a cab back to my parents. Bump, back to reality. Dad was strange. He started to question everything I did again. "Don't do this. Don't do that. When are you leaving?" I couldn't quite put my finger on the change but it's always been the same when I have been away to Hawaii. The tsunami fallout was still rife everywhere however I was finally able to look at a newspaper and see the odd news clip now.

I had been in discussions with my company. They wanted me to go back to the Maldives for a week to sort out the spa, do a report and then go on to my new job in Crete. I was scared to death to go back. Anyway, through my panic I reasoned that it might be a good thing for me to face my fear. Two weeks later I was on a plane flying out to Male via Doha, Qatar, one place I swore I would never want to stay. I arrived in daylight and the familiar scene unfolded. You would never have known there had been such destruction three months earlier. The sun was shining, the sea was deep blue and it was so good to see familiar faces on the speedboat taking us towards our dot in the ocean.

I got to the island and was met by the general manager and assistant manager. It was such a relief to see familiar faces. We hugged and then they took me to my old home! It had been gutted and then restored to nearly all its former glory. How wonderful. I wasn't quite sure how I would sleep and, as it turned out, I hardly slept at all in there, but it was a great gesture.

I was only meant to be there one week, however, I couldn't get a flight out. I had used my return ticket from my holiday following the tsunami, so we agreed that my final return flight back to the UK would be organised from Male. No such luck, it would be four weeks before I would get away again! I had a sneaky feeling it was on purpose!

The island was full of construction workers, worse than before but being stared at this time didn't bother me. I was used to it. A new English teacher had just arrived, so I had female company. She was struggling with the whole male ego thing. The staring and spitting, possessiveness and lack of structure or respect was difficult. You had to earn their respect and behave impeccably. I had a head start and most were incredibly gracious and very happy to see me. We had been through a lot together and they had lived on the island since, some not even having the chance to go home, which was sad.

The company had arranged for some outside trainers to do team building and leadership skills with the staff. As I wasn't officially part of the team and wouldn't be, due to the fact that I was just working there temporarily for one week, I wasn't expected to run the normal operational meetings. My sole purpose was to get into the spa and report on my findings. I had nothing to manage, but I was welcomed and encouraged to join in with the training anyway.

I ended up attending all the trainings and working with my colleagues. For the first time we saw each other in a different light. It was great fun! We worked in the morning, still clearing and keeping the island clean and then attended the training in the afternoon. We would play volleyball in the late afternoon and, after the sun had gone down, a group of us would enjoy a long swim out to a tiny island and back again. In between, I slowly worked my way through the spa, collating information about replacing the damage and stock. I created a comprehensive report to get the spa up to scratch ready for opening.

On the Easter Monday 28th March 2005, exactly three months to the day following the Boxing Day tsunami, I was just about managing to get off to sleep, when at about 11pm came a loud bang at my door. I panicked for a moment, and then let in Anne, the English teacher.

She said, "Now I don't want you to worry, but we have to get to the dive centre. There has been a major earthquake and a tsunami warning."

Well, I did panic. It was the first time ever in my life that I remember reacting like this. I started to tremble, grabbed my suitcase, threw everything in it, locked it and left it on the bed, hoping that if the wave came it wouldn't get to my bed! Well that was my logic, crazy really. I grabbed my laptop and ran with her to the dive centre.

All of us who had experienced the first one, were indignant and scared that this could happen again. We were so vulnerable on this tiny island. I think we were all rattled. Everyone of us had fear written on our faces. We came together with a real sense of camaraderie and strength as we sat and waited this one out. It was the early hours of the morning by the time we went back to our rooms. The time had passed without incident. Anne came back to my room and stayed with me for the night. Neither of us wanted to be alone. I hardly slept a wink.

The next day, we tried to carry on as normal. The trainer decided to give up as we were all so tired. Instead, we played games and then had the rest of the day off. I found it incredible that exactly ninety days after the devastation of Boxing Day, and on another religious day, we should find ourselves reliving the drama and feeling the primal instincts of survival. I should have been in Crete not the Maldives. In a divine way, I was glad to have been stranded on the island for that month. I faced my fear, as we all did and I am sure it helped us all in the long run.

A couple of weeks later, they finally found me a flight out. It was a wrench this time, saying a sad goodbye again to those staying back on the island. I got back to the UK and had a week at home, before flying into a new adventure! I was really looking forward to working and living in Crete. Even though I had visited many other Greek island I had never been to Crete before, it was always one I wanted to visit one day and now that was coming true. How exciting!

My heart and thoughts go out to all those affected by that devastating yet enlightening day in 2004. On the anniversary, I have relived the moment every year so far. The first anniversary, my body went into shock and for 24 hours I felt flu like symptoms and couldn't stop shaking. The second anniversary, I couldn't stop crying for three days. The third anniversary, my mind was in overdrive reliving the visions of that day with horrendous dreams. The fourth anniversary was calm. The fifth anniversary, I was shaking in my core, but it is getting better slowly as the tissue memory of shock and loss slowly heals itself. Christmas time for me is a poignant time for healing. I never suppress what comes up and I ensure I have the space in my life to allow it to surface and release. I am thankful I live happily and normally the rest of the year. May we all live in kindness, love and peace.

WHIRLPOOLS

"Experience is simply the name we give our mistakes"
Oscar Wilde

Island fun

I arrived at Heraklion airport on a day patched with cloud and with a feeling of slight anxiety. The day before I was due to fly I had heard that the family owners I would be working with had expected me a month earlier. I had no idea that my company had been stalling getting me there because of the situation in the Maldives, which meant I had no idea what I was walking into. The feeling of trepidation increased.

I needn't have worried. It was Greek Easter weekend, a perfect time to arrive. In amongst the frivolity and festivities everyone was on a high. Greek Easter is traditionally the start of the working season and everyone was gearing up to receive the first tourists of the year.

I was given a royal greeting, a maze of different faces, all grinning from ear to ear. I suspected because of too much ouzo! I was escorted to what was to become my home for the duration of my stay, a wonderful little bungalow in the gardens of a hotel with a view out to the ocean. A far cry from my initial room in the Maldives that was tiny and dark.

I enjoyed the bungalow, tucked away in a corner of a beautiful rustic Cretan style hotel. It had stunning views and its own pool. The Greek hospitality stood up to its reputation and I felt very welcome. They had specially installed an internet connection so I could communicate out of hours with my head office in Thailand. It seemed they couldn't do enough for me.

I attended the festivities, getting to feel the vibe. During the first two days I started to explore my surroundings and get familiarised with the job at hand. The family owned three hotels, all located in a beautiful region of the island which was surrounded by rolling hills and sheltered in a long bay. Each hotel offered a different standard of accommodation and facilities and each had its own spa. In addition, within the biggest of the three hotels, they were building a huge spa which would replace the smaller units. The main spa was due to open the following year. My job was to set up the operation and open the three spas, which included recruiting a team for each, training them in standards of operation and in the treatments to be given by the therapists, a big job in itself. In addition, I was to oversee the new build to ensure the works were being built to the standards of our company, whilst embracing its environmentally sound ethos.

On my first free evening a sense of nostalgia enveloped me. Greece was familiar territory, which was definitely in my favour. I decided to walk the two miles into the village and took the path along the sea front where I came across a row of tavernas. I chose one I liked the look of and sat watching the sunset. It was very reminiscent of the Shirley Valentine film, sitting on my own with a view out to sea. It was a clear, cool evening. I couldn't wait to savour a Greek salad and Kalamari, my favourite Greek dishes and, of course, sample the ouzo. This was such a contrast to the restrictions of being a woman in the Maldives where if I had eaten and drunk alcohol in a restaurant on my own, I would have been locked up! After one ouzo, which went straight to my head, I felt free and relaxed for the first time in a long while.

The holiday season was due to open and the new spa was just a shell of walls and concrete. It was a huge project. I quickly found out that my personal boundaries were to be tested once again. After a promising start, I realised that in their eyes I was their property with 24/7 access. I was also suffering from post traumatic stress syndrome as it was still only four months since the tsunami. I began to have dreams about a big wave hitting the island of Crete and surviving the wave that swallowed up the land. In the dream, there was a small group of us and I literally dragged people up a steep hill. An immense strength took over inside me as the survival instinct kicked in. In the dream we didn't look back until we could go no further. As we reached high ground, we turned round to a view of turmoil, dead bloated bodies and debris. The dreams were most disturbing and very real. It gave me an uneasy feeling of being here on another island, vulnerable.

I later made the connection, that when the volcano erupted on Santorini some three thousand years before, it had created a huge tsunami wave which hit Crete, devastating the Minoan civilisation. Perhaps I was tapping into a part of reality that the land held in its memory from a long time ago.

I put up a brave front, but I was still particularly sensitive and fearful at times, so I became very protective over my time and became more and more insular. I began to stand my ground and ensured that I structured my days according to the needs of the business. I didn't want to be pulled from pillar to post according to the volatility of the family dynamic around me. I was here to do a job, but not at the expense of my own integrity.

The manager was a strong Greek woman and she was driven and competitive. Slowly the games began. I love the Greeks, but boy do they play emotional games. The family involved in the project created its own drama as each individual had a role to play, but they pushed each others buttons to boiling point. I was very often a witness to the high and lows of rows and gossip. It was incredible and, actually sometimes, so farcical that I would end up laughing in the middle of it. This normally resulted in a few smiles as they knew exactly what they were doing.

Besides all the politics and family rows, I was enjoying a sense of freedom. When I finished work I would take the opportunity and walk into the village. The weather was getting warmer and I loved the beautiful spring time flowers and the soft fragrance in the air. My route into the village took me past a rental car business, which two brothers owned and ran. I would stop and have a quick chat to pass the time of day and they would sometimes get me to jump on the back of their motorbike and take me the rest of the way. They became my protectors of sorts. I didn't tell them much about what I was doing and they weren't really interested, just happy to talk about the local gossip and events happening in the country.

Love's dream

Life began to slow down. Work was intense, with long hours, but it didn't matter as I could walk out in the warm evening under the stars and feel safe again. I had been in Crete for about two and a half months, I guess, when the 'boys,' as I called them, from the rent-a-car business started to invite me out for a drink. I kept saying no. Then one day, the older brother asked me what I was doing that night.

I said, "I'm going for something to eat, then home to sleep."

In his Greek accent, he said, "Join me and the lads for a drink. Go on."

Much to my better judgement, I gave in and said "Okay."

I went for something to eat and it was about eleven o'clock when I left the taverna. I decided to go and have a drink with the lads. When I turned the corner, I saw Adonis sat with another man. I was slightly relieved as I thought that when he had said the lads he might have meant a big group. My plan had been to say hello and then give some excuse to leave.

It was a relaxed evening as we sat outside and started chatting. His friends' name was David. Half Dutch and half German, he had lived nearly all of his life in Greece. David was fluent in English, Greek, German and Dutch. He was very much accepted in the community as a Greek and was a best friend of the brothers. David was over six foot talk, slim, with a handsome tanned face and slightly thinning hair, but I liked the look of him and we ended up having a wonderful easy going time. He offered me a lift back to my hotel and we said goodbye. I let it all go, grateful for a nice time and thinking I didn't want to get involved with anyone, no matter how lonely I felt.

A couple of days passed and I received a call from David at work. He asked me out for a meal that evening. I wasn't sure what to say but my heart started jumping and I felt excited so I accepted. The evening was truly magical. He picked me up on the back of his motorbike. I held on for dear life as we found our way to a typical Greek taverna on a hillside overlooking the town. The night sky was as clear as a bell and the moon was full. We chatted for ages, left the taverna and went to a bar located over the water. It was all so romantic.

Safe and comfortable with David, I said to him I wanted to take him to a special place I had found over the other side of the bay and would he mind going? We drove down a dirt track to the other side of a hill. It was here that I would spend some of my days off in quiet contemplation. There was a tiny church with an ancient olive tree in its grounds. The stars and the moon were so bright that night. As we parked up, it was dead quiet. I turned around and in the bushes, not far away, was a huge owl. It stared at us both. We watched for a while, and then it turned and flew away; an ominous sign perhaps?

I guided David into the grounds and we sat in silence by the olive tree for a while. It was quiet, peaceful and calm watching the night sky. After a while, we stood up to go back and for a moment held each other looking up towards the stars. All of a sudden, as if something had frightened him, he said, "Oh my God! I feel like the top of my head has been blown apart. We have to go, I can't deal with this." A strange thing to say I thought, but I didn't pursue it.

The next day we met up and he said he had never experienced anything like it before. He said that it was as if he couldn't comprehend the vastness of time and space and that his head was going to explode. He said he felt different. I then realised that the place I had taken him was a powerful spot, normal for me, however for David a new experience. Maybe I should have waited until I had known him a bit better before taking him to a place like that.

I thought this experience might frighten him away, but it didn't. After that he wanted to see me more and more. I was a little wary as he was on the rebound from his wife of ten years. Apparently, she had decided she no longer loved him and wanted him out of the house. Well, that was his story. Knowing that there were always two sides to a story, I just kept my own counsel and maintained this in perspective as much as I could. I could see he missed his two boys and it was evident that he was suppressing his feelings about the break up. David had thrown himself into work and was doing two jobs. Our time together would be late in the evening, actually too late for me, and on a Sunday afternoon. I knew he wasn't ready to be in a relationship, yet I was lonely and he was adamant that he wanted a different life to the one he was living so I stuck around. I still wasn't quite myself and I loved the fact that I could be close to someone. I was still dealing with the aftermath of my own stuff and feeling lonely, his strong arms around me made me feel safe. It also stirred up the romantic energy inside of me. It had been such a long time since anyone had really taken an interest in me.

So, it was during this time of neediness that I slipped back into an old pattern. Forgetting my own needs, I began to get really tired, following his daily routine rather than mine. I would wait for him to collect me late at night so that we could snatch some time together. Then I would get up early to start my days' work. My boundaries had all but disappeared again and I found myself moulding into his way of life. He drank a lot and smoked which was something I abhorred. I started to join him for a drink after work, which I knew was not good for me. I simply enjoyed the attention, albeit distorted, without any real grounded connection to my own truth. So I let it go and continued to get more and more tired. I started to feel unwell and disgruntled with work.

Out of the blue, I received an email from the coffee shop guy that I had met a couple of years previously in the UK. The one I really liked but was married. Well, he was finally going through a divorce and wondered where I was and what I was up to. Talk about timing! As my relationship with David was in its early stage, I exchanged a few friendly emails with him, telling him where I was and telling him that I was dating someone. I realised he also wasn't in a good space to start up something even if that's what he wanted.

He had an awful long way to go before he would be really available to someone else and I wasn't prepared to give up what I had started here just yet. We agreed to keep in touch and wished each other well. I was yet again amazed at the synchronicity of the timing. Perhaps this was a sign for me to let go of David, as although I loved our connection, the whole way of living wasn't right for me and we were still in the lust stage so I couldn't quite find the clarity to get to the truth. Another lesson was emerging.

After we had been dating for about five months, I had to go back to the UK for a three week period for work. I had also booked a trip to Hawaii at the beginning of the season to ensure that I didn't do what I did in the Maldives and not take a break. It had been planned so that I could go straight from the UK to Hawaii on leave. David didn't like the idea of me going at all. It appeared that I acted as some sort of calming drug for him, or so he said. I started to worry about his state of mind as he kept on saying that he didn't know how long he could go on like this. When I asked what he meant, he couldn't explain. My rescuer instincts took over from all reason and I absorbed my time outside of work on him. Deep down I knew this wasn't right. I knew also I was really far away from my truth again, entangled emotionally, both with him and with myself. How could I possibly choose a different path?

With deep anxiety, I left to go the UK. It was autumn time, one of my favourite seasons. All this time David was on my mind, absorbing any spare thinking and feeling time that I had. I had no strength to separate my energy at this time and I was exhausted.

It didn't help that when he called, all he would focus on was how he missed me and could I get back soon. I began to think, "Should I go to Hawaii, or should I spend my holiday in Crete and be near David?" His neediness was a drug. I knew I wanted to be doing what I was doing and equally, really wanted my holiday. Thankfully, he started to become calmer as the tourist season got quieter and he had more time to rest. My feelings of wanting to go and save him lessened as we talked on the phone almost daily. These calls were a drain in themselves as I came to realise. I completed my work in the UK and I got on a flight to Hawaii.

Soul connection

I immediately felt at home again arriving into Kahului, Maui for the second time that year. I felt incredibly thankful that I was able to afford to come again and so soon. In the back of my mind however was David. How was he? Was he okay? It felt like I was his mother worrying about his state of health. Actually it was his drinking that was the problem.

Anyhow, I continued to enjoy my time and met up with some old friends, including Nicole. This trip was different. I didn't feel the need to do any deep work. This was purely restoration time. I spent a week on Maui then a week on Kaua'i. It was in Kaua'i that I felt pangs of panic about David. He would tell me he couldn't cope without me and his heart physically hurt. I told him to get it checked out. Then I would think, "Is he doing this on purpose because he knows I care?" It was a real test for me. Should I come home early I would ask him? "No," he would say. "I'll be alright, but come home soon as I don't know how I can go on like this." Now, I wasn't sure what he meant here either. Did he mean to stay with me or was he having a breakdown of some sort? I was confused. Then, all of a sudden he said he had something special for me on my return. I was allowing my emotions to be tossed around in a whirlpool. Déjà vu, here we go again.

Hawaii had given me some of my strength back. My energy was stronger and I felt a sense of resolve. I was kind of excited about my return. By the time I started the long journey back, David had calmed down a lot more. I eventually landed back in Crete after about six weeks away. Everything was quiet in the village. The tourists had left for the season giving the place a completely different feel. David met me at the airport and he seemed alright. He drove me home and gave me the surprise. It was a gold ring with initials engraved on it, not an engagement ring, but a family ring. It was not the first one he had given as I was to find out later. Both his ex-wives had received one. Yes, I did say two ex-wives! David had three children in all. I was not one to be ungrateful and it was a lovely gesture however, it didn't entirely make me feel very special. It felt like I became one of his harem!

Turning point

I got back to work and we continued seeing each other, but something had changed. I sensed a shift. Was it in me, him or both of us? Perhaps he was depressed, I thought. It would have been quite understandable as he was winding down from such a busy time, or was it me. But no, he didn't really seem interested in the same way as before. This was reminiscent of when my ex-husband came back from Beirut. Deep down I knew something wasn't right as once again I knew, right from the beginning, that I wasn't being fulfilled. He would say the right things to me, but his actions and my intuition was telling me different. Desperately wanting to get away from the island, he wanted to leave and work somewhere else in the world and he was even prepared to leave his kids.

The project I had been working on in Crete had come to an end for now. I was asked to go back to the Maldives again for an interim period, until they could sort out a replacement. I couldn't bear the thought of not being with David. I had another choice to make, my career or a relationship.

David and I decided to start a new life away from Greece altogether and we came back to the UK. I had left the company that I worked for and decided that I would set up practise again and do some consultancy work on the side. Before that was Christmas and New Year. We left Greece just before Christmas and went to spend the festivities with his parents in Germany. It was the first time he had been with his family for years. I was very honoured to be a part of that reunion. They were lovely people. We were to spend New Year with my parents.

On Christmas night, I began to feel extremely unwell. I was sweating, shivering and generally feeling like my whole body was going to explode with pain. I offered my apologies and went to bed. David came in to check on me and I was completely cold and shivering, even though I was covered in blankets. This was the first anniversary of the tsunami and I had gone into shock. It lasted for about a day before I started to feel better. After Christmas, we returned from Germany to the UK and spent a lovely New Year with my parents.

Back in the UK, David found a job straight away in a hotel. It was long hours again, the same pattern as back in Greece. I set up my own practise and worked part time as a consultant. For me, life was good. I really enjoyed my clients and the contrast of working in the business world. I was doing very well. We rented a lovely apartment near to the beach and it seemed we had everything we needed. My own boundaries strengthened. David didn't seem to care about anything except his drink and working all hours. He said he missed his kids, but wouldn't do anything about going to see them. I couldn't understand this. He constantly moaned about his work, but was not prepared to do anything about that either. I came to the conclusion that he loved being the way he was and doing what he did and it was his choice to live in that way.

I was very content with my professional life so I had the best of both worlds. My relationship wasn't great. I was constantly being governed by David's moods. He still drank too much and I knew it affected him. His behaviour was inconsistent. Just subtle things that happened, he would say one thing and do another. I realised this and accepted the situation, not willing to upset the applecart or ready to let it go. A part of me still held on to the special moments of our potential when we first met. It was the potential of the relationship that I fell for. David, I was to find out, was never going to wake up, and why should I expect him to? It was his choice not mine.

It got to a crunch point when he announced that he didn't like this country anymore and wanted to work somewhere else. He had no thought for the life we had built up and was without any thought for my work. It seemed surreal. After all our conversations about life and expressing ourselves, actually it wasn't like that at all. Instead of me letting him go, and him letting me go, to go our separate ways, I tried to fix the situation again. All the time I knew this wasn't right. It was easier for me to find work in my line of business overseas so I got a job back with my old company. The plan was that I would go to a job in the Middle East and he would follow in three months, as my company had offered him a job in a new hotel that they were refurbishing in Jordan. I was to be the pre-opening manager for a spa project there. Hadn't I been and done this before?

I did say, in one of my earlier chapters, that it takes time to change behaviours! My instincts knew that this was all wrong and this was a perfect example of me not wanting to let go of a distorted reality. I knew when I came back from Hawaii on holiday, that there was a change in our relationship. My needs would never be satisfied by this man, yet I chose to continue accepting less than what I was worthy of. He was a good guy underneath it all, but was not, at this time, able to make that transition in his own life. We simply were on different paths.

Anyway, realising deep down that this was wrong and that I was repeating an old pattern, I still went into overdrive, trying to solve the problem. Mentally, this all sounded like a perfect plan for us both, except that I wasn't enamoured about going to the Middle East region and I had never had a pull to go there. A big part of me was also very reluctant and sad to give up what I had built in my professional life, let alone the clients that I had built up a relationship with. However, I thought our relationship was more important and although he drank too much and was secretive, I still thought I had a strong connection with this man, a connection that filled a deep need inside of me. David couldn't wait to get going on this new plan either.

I was holding onto the magic that we shared in the beginning, that spark of potential I saw in him. In reality, he actually couldn't give me anything in return and deep down I knew I was accepting less than was good for me. Three months later, I was on a plane to Qatar. Work plans had changed and I was to be interim director in a newly opened Spa in Doha for a month before going to my base in Jordan. Doha was a place I vowed I would never like to work. Little did I know that would be the last I saw of David. My trusted instinct and guidance were giving me every sign they could muster, to let David go, but I still chose to go headlong into, what was to become, a tumultuous eight months. What an experience!

Arabian nights

Qatar, Doha, on the edge of the Arabian Sea, is a city built up from the barren and dusty desert. It was the next Dubai and a city under a siege of construction. Every street had building work and huge areas excavated ready to build yet another high rise, shiny, smart looking building.

It was hot, very hot. I was taken to my apartment and shown into a smart and huge space. It had all that was required. The spa I was to direct for the next month, was a fifteen minute walk away. The walk was hellish, along a main road where cars would scream along at an amazing speed, driven by drivers not particularly aware, only seeing what was in front of them. Every so often, they would toot. It was very annoying. It was because I was female. The men would stare and glare and tut under their breath. It was most unnerving and oddly made me feel angry. What the hell am I doing here?

The spa was huge, built like a traditional Qatari village and quite unique. I had a team of sixty staff to manage and hold together like glue. Many things happened during my time there. The goal posts were changed as my company put off recruiting a new director until after Christmas so I was to stay until then. I was not happy. I felt trapped. This was not what I had signed up for. To top it all, immigration had full control over whether you could leave or not. I just couldn't up and walk out. To get out of the country your exit visa would have to be granted by the Immigration Office, which meant your passport was kept by the company where I worked. It was a horrible feeling of imprisonment.

In the interim, I had an appointment to meet the owners of the project in Jordan. I had to go over for a week. It was traumatic waiting for my passport to come back from Immigration with the exit visa. I didn't get my passport back until one hour before my flight to Amman.

Jordan was very different. The airport was like something out of the 1970's, the men wore black leather jackets and everyone smoked. I was picked up from the airport and driven along well maintained roads for about ten minutes then, all of a sudden, the roads changed to pot holed tracks. There didn't seem to be any rules about what side of the road you drove on! It was all a bit hit and miss. What an adventure. It was about an hour's drive, along and down into the Dead Sea region, where we travelled down a steep road deep in to a valley below where the hotel and spa was located.

I could breathe here. We were four hundred metres below sea level and the oxygen was rich. Sleep was heavenly. The hotel was still open for guests but due to close for refurbishment in the New Year. We drove down into a national park area, and passed a ridge of hot springs. It was a tremendous sight. At night, all through the valley and across the Dead Sea, you could see the bright lights of Jerusalem. This is what I signed up for. I could see myself here and I felt good. The people were friendly and welcoming. I met the owners and walked round the newly built spa to get a feel for what was required and enjoyed a fabulous week. It was a shame I had to go back to Doha.

What kept me going was David coming out after Christmas. We would be together in Jordan, where my heart was yearning to go. Two weeks before Christmas when I'd been away for about six weeks, David suddenly stopped communicating with me. I couldn't get out of him why he stopped, in the end, I emailed and asked him to please tell me what was going on for him. I was shocked at what came back. "I'm not coming out to Jordan. I'm not coming to see you. I don't love you anymore and we are finished."

It was like being hit with a steam roller. He had told me just before I had left that he loved me and wanted to be with me for the rest of our lives. I was willing to compromise to make this happen. All sorts of emotions and questions bubbled up, anger, betrayal, concern. Why? What had changed? I couldn't make sense of this at all, although deep down, I knew. However, on the surface I became incensed. There were no answers forthcoming and he couldn't explain it. He just said that he wanted to go back to Greece, where for him life had been hell or so he had said. In reality, he didn't go back to Greece and during the next few months he stayed put in the UK, so there must have been another reason but I never found out what it was.

I was hurting. I felt he had deceived me. Why now? If he was unsure, why not do this before I gave up everything? In reality, I had deceived myself. Knowing this still didn't take away the pain as I came to realise he actually knew this would happen. In his selfishness, he let me give up everything, fly to a strange land and then dumped me. How cowardly is that? I was raging inside. A year earlier, I had given up a job opportunity in Hawaii to be with David. He didn't want me to go and he couldn't come with me, so I chose him over my career and my dream. My choices were blinded by the possibility of finding a truthful love. This man had so much potential in that respect, but it seemed not with me.

When I had started seeing David, I promised myself that I would express myself to him, not let things boil inside as I did with my ex husband and I asked him if he could find it in himself to try to do the same, no matter how difficult it may be. If something wasn't right we should express it, that way we both had a choice. I know I upheld that promise to myself, however, I guess it was too much for him. There was much hidden beneath the surface that was too conflicting for him to reason with. I recognised my part in all of this as I realised he wasn't on the same page as me and there was never going to be the relationship that I was ready for with this man.

My guidance had given me every opportunity to let this relationship go. In hindsight the time leading up to leaving Crete should have been the time that I really listened to the signs and taken a back step in the relationship. However, this whole period in my life gave me another strengthening realisation and an opportunity to really ground in my boundaries and not accept anything less than I deserved and am worthy of.

Lucky escape

Anyway, here I was still in the Middle East, alone and feeling sorry for myself. I spent time with a colleague and his partner, who had both been stranded in Doha for Christmas due to passport problems. Together we enjoyed a Christmas lunch buffet in one of hotels and collaborated in putting relationships and the worlds to right. To top it all, the Qatarian Government had put a freeze on recruitment and we were desperate for staff which meant I had to stay longer.

I cried a lot during this time. It was painful to be dumped like that, so far away from friends and family in a hostile country. Especially as all the plans had been made for him rather than me. Feeling sorry for myself and giving myself a hard time, I felt I was being tossed around again and I knew I done this all before.

I had called Mum and Dad on Christmas Day. Mum said Dad wasn't well and he hadn't had anything to eat. I said he should go to the hospital. Dad came on the phone, and as normal, played the whole thing down saying he was alright.

Boxing Day arrived and I tried to call home. No answer. "Strange." I thought, as I tried more times throughout the day. I began to worry, as Mum and Dad didn't go out on Boxing Day. I called my brother. He said, "Oh yes, Dad was taken into hospital." I asked him for the number to the hospital, so I could call to find out what's happening. All my sorrows paled into insignificance now as I fretted about Dad. He had kidney failure and had kept it a secret. He had been suffering in pain for months now.

The next few days were awful. I was constantly trying to get sense out of mother, who couldn't remember all the details, bless her. She was worried. It wasn't normal for Dad to be ill, you see. Dad's friends rallied round, my brother did his best to support Mum, and I was miles away stuck in a country that I never wanted to be in. I was in a deep whirlpool of emotional trauma. How much more could I take?!

Dad ended up being in hospital for just under three months. He was diagnosed with bladder cancer and his bladder was removed eventually. He was lucky to be alive. I managed to get leave and go home before he had the operation and was thankful to see him. What a change. He had lost so much weight and looked frail. Mum managed the best she could and I stayed on leave for a while. Then, my sister came over from Ireland and my brother stayed too. In between time, friends helped with the dog walking and taking Mum to the hospital to see Dad.

It was a horrible time. I had battles going on inside me as to whether or not give it all up and go home to look after Mum whilst Dad was in hospital. All the time, I had the huge responsibility of looking after a team of people and trying to recruit my replacement so that I could go. I also had no home of my own to go back to.

The sorrow of another relationship down the pan left me depressed, stressed and desperately unhappy with my lot, but I didn't have the inner strength to do something about it until my replacement arrived.

The new spa director and I had a three week handover, before I was due to leave for Jordan where I should have been in the first place. First, I wanted to go home to see Dad come out of hospital. In the meantime, I visited Jordan and saw where I would be living and realised I would be extremely vulnerable there. Anyway, what the hell was I doing with my life? David wouldn't be joining me and I was thousands of miles away from my friends. Why was I here?! I decided I'd had enough of messing around and pleasing other people and handed in my notice. I was done with this kind of life.

Not knowing where or what I was going to do, I started searching for a job in the UK. Remarkably there was a great job going near to where I wanted to live. Not many opportunities became available in that particular neck of the woods, or at that level, so it seemed like it was heaven sent. I got through the telephone interview and made arrangements to meet them on my return to the UK. It was a director's role in a very prestigious company.

Dad had just come out of hospital after struggling against all odds. He had contracted two hospital super bugs during his time following the operation as well as dealing with the cancer. I got the job! Perfect timing and I was just where I should be.

I found a lovely place to live with a sea view and after a while of being back in the UK, I was able to make sense of the choices I had made over the past couple of years between David and my career. I had compromised myself in many ways again however, this time, I had been conscious of my choices, just not strong enough emotionally to carry through. Although it was an extreme time in the Middle East, I am grateful that it enabled me to see clear priorities eventually. Life in the mists of the distortion of everyday living, once the emotion has cleared and forgiveness realised, is an exciting challenge. I realised all experiences are to be embraced and loved.

I met up with David when I came back to the UK eight months later. He was still there and still living the same drama. I gave him back his belongings that had been stored for him, wished him luck and said goodbye with a smile on my face. A couple of weeks later a friend told me he went back to Greece.

Yet again I felt like I had cleared much baggage, another layer of stuff as I had unconsciously been attracted to situations in order to allow myself to grow, become clearer and more at peace. This chapter of my life was like being in a whirlpool, playing out many a life times of experience. Strangely, I felt calm about the next adventure to come.

INFINITE DEEP WATERS OF LIFE

*"And in the end, it's not the years in your life that count.
It's the life in your years"*
Abraham Lincoln

Calm before the storm

Dad was doing well considering what he had gone through and continued to get stronger after his major surgery. The following summer, after his stay in hospital, I was able to visit my parents more often. I saw him struggle to walk, first around the house, then slowly his determination to improve against all odds. He started to walk the dog, a little way at a time. Our little schnauzer loved it! She had her Dad back. She would dance around and spin on the spot when there was any sense of him moving out of his chair to go to the kitchen to get her lead. The surgery had given him a lifeline, for how long we had no idea. He had decided against chemotherapy or any other type of treatment at this stage, believing that treatment would make his quality of life unbearable for a while, with no guarantee of a quality of life afterwards. He preferred instead to get back to some sort of fitness through his own efforts. The operation had removed a large proportion of the cancer and he was adjusting to life with a urostomy stoma.

We all honoured his choice and were grateful to still have him with us. I spent a year in my job and realised that I wanted a quality of life too again, so I let go of the security and started up a business on my own. I loved it, found peace in what I was doing and time to write, laugh, play and find solitude – which I craved. I began to build on my inner strength, knowing this time was precious; it was like the calm before the storm, as I knew difficult times were to come. The universe was looking after me yet again, knowing at one level the next experience would be something I had always dreaded, yet now I felt ready for. Dad was slowly beginning to deteriorate, the cancer had started to spread and rage inside his body.

It was to be another year before I finally went back to stay with my parents full time, giving up my business to see through this 'phase' with my family. During that year, my father, proud as ever would ask me every so often if I was happy where I was and hinting strongly that mother would need some help as he got weaker. The question was, would I consider coming back to live in with them during this time. It was a big decision for me, as it would mean letting go of a lifestyle that I really enjoyed and a place that I loved to be. It would also mean going back into a toxic family dynamic, which I had dealt with many years ago and I wasn't sure if I had the courage to deal with again.

However, I felt a huge obligation and a real 'pull' that this was a something I simply had to do. It felt like I had made a contract with my father at some point in the past, to help him through his last months of life - the tug was immense. I began to sense he was almost desperate for me to be at home with them. I rationalised that as Mother had never had to take care of Dad, I guess he was fearful of how she would react when things got worse.

So, what occurred next was magical. The timing of what was to come was perfectly masterminded on all levels. It took me three months exactly to move back to the family home. Within two weeks of me moving back, Dad stopped walking the dog – it was simply too much. Weakness started to take over, I took over his responsibilities in the house, as mother wouldn't or couldn't at this stage.

However, the battles started with my mother. Without me knowing, she had made it clear to Dad before I came that she didn't want me living with them; however, Dad had been insistent, saying I would be there to support her not him. It could have been my brother or sister, but they had families of their own. In his mind that is what he wanted, for me to take care of mother, so he could relinquish that responsibility and know that mother would be taken care of. In the end he found that the most difficult, to let go of mother as he stilled worried about her.

So I found myself in the same house I was born in. It was like going back to childhood. Mothers jealousy was overbearing, her moods indescribable. Yet for my Dad her moods were completely normal as he had lived with this for years. Reluctantly she began to recognise the value of having another 'adult' in the house, as Dad started the process of letting go.

In the midst of all the emotional and mental distortion at home it was work that was to bring clarity and light to my world. A perfect job came up for me, very near to the family home. It gave me the means and time to do what I needed to do for my family. I really enjoyed my time at work, a respite from the grey moods of mother and the pain of watching Dad slowly deteriorate. I sometimes behaved just as badly back to my mother. I couldn't help it, it was enormously upsetting to see Dad getting weaker by the day, his faculties slowing diminishing physically, his body starting to let go and be consumed by the disease. I couldn't understand her behaviour. In hindsight I can only guess, she was fearful of losing him and lashed out. However I really do not know to this day what drove her, as in truth she was like this normally and had been all the time I had known her.

The months went by, mother's moods and rages were wearing both him and me down now. He no longer had the strength and I could now see it clearly. Her moods would fluctuate. Quiet anger and hate being directed at him and then me and then both of us. Sometimes, it became unbearable and I wanted to get away from it all. The internal stress within me was pushing my boundaries to an extreme. There were moments of delight, as suddenly she would wake up and obviously feel good and be okay for a day or two, if we were lucky this would last a couple of weeks. Then a look from me or the way I said something and her mind switched, interpreting it in a way that would trigger her off again and we would be back to normal.

I really dug deep to be with it and was determined for Dad's sake to hang around. He wouldn't hear of me going, as it appeared on the surface that me being there made her worse. Dad denied this and said it was 'normal behaviour.' Sometimes when it was bad, we would talk about the situation. One day he asked me if I thought mother really loved him – I couldn't honestly answer, as I actually didn't really know. All I did know that she had always been this way and I had known no different throughout my life. Dad would blame it on the many different tablets she took, rather than see his wife as someone with a choice. I had seen her change her behaviour in a flash when required in front of other people and depending on what was going on in her mind. I knew there really was an underlying strength, with an ability to change. She was also stuck in a pattern of destruction, in this case, affecting those around her.

The weeks and months passed and Dad knew exactly what was going on. He was still in control of his mind and I felt incredibly proud of the way he was handling the whole situation. Very matter of fact about what was to come, not fearful, just accepting. We spent time sorting out his affairs and easing his mind by ensuring everything was in place for mother when he was no longer around. We discussed the illness openly with the family doctor and the nurses, he didn't hide anything. We organised a family get together to discuss what was to come and to plan his funeral. We discussed every aspect of his palliative care and gave our opinion when asked for. For the first time ever, he allowed me to massage his legs and help out physically, even though it was to such a small degree – I felt thankful and grateful for that opportunity.

The months went on, the summer was lovely and Dad enjoyed some of the time sitting out in the garden, watching the clouds and listening to the birds sing then falling asleep. His mind was still relatively sharp, his body was decaying. It was so cruel. I am not sure what is worse, the body slowly decaying first or the mind going first – both are equally challenging for those around watching it happen. At least we could have a conversation with him. The end of August came and Dad was getting weaker, using a walking stick to get up in the morning and struggle into the lounge. The carers were coming in to help him wash, which gave him someone to boss around, much aligned to his character!

Still incredibly proud, he would try and do everything himself, even though it was extremely difficult to do the most simplest of actions. The hospital bed was delivered, as he expressed most passionately that he wanted to pass away at home and was paranoid about going into hospital. Both mum and I had strict instructions that whatever happened he was not to be taken to hospital and paramedics were to deal with the condition at home, even if that meant him dying.

For the first time mother started to take care of Dad, the reality of the situation kicking in at last, she cooked, cleaned and waited on him, feeling for the first time capable of doing something good. I began to see another side of her and actually felt respect that she rose above her pain to do this. It took the pressure off me as I found myself less worried when I was at work, knowing she was doing her best when I wasn't there.

Endings are dear

Beginning of September, the leaves on the trees were beginning to change colour, Autumn was emerging. Dad was now sleeping in the hospital bed in the lounge, where he could watch and control the television. At least that was something he could still do! It was getting increasingly difficult for him to get up out of bed into the wheelchair to be taken to the toilet. His biggest fear was the toilet issue, what and how would he go to the toilet once he could no longer get out of bed. This worried him. We got all the help we could. He had an urostomy bag and that part was easy to manage. It was the other part that created huge stress on him. In the end once he simply could not get up, he stopped eating, I think it was fear of messing the bed and became really weak.

Becoming delusional, he would only sip water. In between episodes of confusion he seemed normal, chatting away. I had a feeling I shouldn't go into work, but I went in anyway not feeling good about it and decided to leave to go home at lunchtime. I was glad I did, as the nurses were there. Dad was putting on a brave face. He was relatively cheery when they left. The nurses said to call out the emergency nurse if he needed anything that night. I think they knew he didn't have long.

I went to bed as normal, said good night to Dad, saying I loved him. I had been listening for his gurgling breathing for months now, and I kept the bedroom door open, so I could hear what was going on. This night I heard more than the heavy breathing, I thought I heard him talking. I got up. It was midnight and pitch black. He was talking loudly saying, "Turn the bloody light on - what's going on here?"

Through the darkness I said, "Dad it's me Jane, I am going to turn on your table light."

At that point he became calm and started almost talking normally to me. I asked him what was going on and he said, "I don't like this, my mind is going all over the place."

What are you seeing Dad I asked, "All sorts of things, I cannot stand this anymore"

"Shall I call the emergency nurse Dad?"

"Yes."

In amongst the sad reality of the situation, the next hour was something out of a comedy sketch. I called the emergency district nurse. In the meantime, I thought I should wake mother, as I knew she would be upset with me for dealing with this without her. I went into her bedroom, she was snoring loudly and not responding to my voice or a kind of gentle nudging. I knew she took strong sleeping tablets, so I decided to leave her sleeping rather than waking her from such a drugged up deep sleep. I went and sat with Dad and we chatted for a while.

Mother must have woken up as the next thing she came into the lounge disorientated, unsteady on her feet and ranting, "What's up with Dad, what's happening and why am I up?" I sat her down in the chair. She was like a little girl, wondering what was going on. The nurses arrived and were unsure of who the patient was! Both parents were delirious!

Dad, being a proper gentlemen, shook the nurse's hand, who informed him he would give an injection to help him sleep. As the nurse was about to give the injection, Dad shouted to me, "Jane, check it's the right one." Even in his state of delirium he was conscious enough to know what was going on and also still fearful for his life. Survival mode was still at work. Little did I know that was the last time I would see him consciously alive.

After the nurses left, I put mother back to bed and sat up with Dad for a while, listening to his now less gurgly but heavier breathing. He seemed at peace and sleeping , so after a while I went back to bed, left all the doors open to listen out. It must have been early hours in the morning when I fell asleep.

I woke up with a start. I couldn't hear Dad's heavy breathing, just a gurgling. I panicked and ran into the lounge. I found him slumped to one side with dried dark fluid coming out of the side of his mouth. He had manoeuvred himself to tilt his head to the side to where the rubbish bin was placed by the bed. Whatever was coming up, came out of the side of his mouth and ran out and down, rather than choking him. He was obviously in a semi conscious state and not able to move his limbs himself, but somehow he had moved in the night to ensure he didn't choke. I cleaned his mouth up and moistened his lips. He murmured every now and then when I asked him a question. It was very sad.

Mum got up and was concerned and started to berate herself for taking the sleeping tablets as she realised what had happened, but simply could not respond in the state she was in. I called the nurses' number and shortly after they turned up, just as Dad was beginning to bleed from his mouth again. They immediately took charge of the situation, making Dad comfortable and giving him a morphine injection. Throughout Dad's illness he had insisted he wasn't in pain, now we couldn't really tell.

It was on a sunny autumn day at the end of September, the last hours and minutes of life for our beloved father were fading away. I called my brother and told him to get home from work as soon as possible. I called my sister in Ireland who was able to say her piece to him over the phone, even though he couldn't respond, he heard her. Mother sat by his side, it was a lovely sight as she stroked his hair and he smiled lightly. My brother arrived just in time, the three of us sat around his bed until he took his last breath of life.

Survival mode

I went into overdrive or perhaps it was survival mode. Organising the funeral kept me busy. My mother, brother and sister allowed me that privilege. Mother didn't want to arrange the funeral, in fact she didn't want to say anything good about Dad, only that he hadn't been a good husband! However, we guessed that may be just her reaction. She started to become jealous again, so we tried to include her as much as possible. None of us were impressed, as the last three weeks of Dad's life she was a different person, actually looking after him and being pleasant, now where had that women gone?

Both my brother and sister stayed in the family home during the week leading up to the funeral. It was a very special bonding time for the three of us and particularly a great support for me. My sister and I really resonated for the first time. We were candid about both our relationships with Dad and Mum. We realised that we had been pitted against each other when we were young. Mother had made sure that my sister and I would dislike each other, not conscious of her actions. Mother would tell her that I was Dad's favourite and he didn't really like her.

I now knew my sister had a hard time growing up too, this confirmed that we really were kindred spirit in the same torrent of distorted truths. When Mother was on a 'downer' she was never able to distinguish what was truth and what was fantasy – this was the sad thing. All three of us suffered.

For the first time ever my sister honoured and thanked me for taking care of our parents during this time, knowing how difficult it had been. She too has been deeply affected by our family dynamic, yet now is a lovely human being and able to see clearly what our lives were really about. It is a blessing that during Dad's illness, it bought us together and all the old hurts had been forgiven once and for all.

We realised that the truth is never far from the surface and mother had a choice to make in terms of how she wanted to behave going forward. I was to stay with her for the near future, to help her settle into different way of life after Dad. The day of the funeral, she decided to lay down her weapon and told me directly she wanted to get along with me and so she changed, just like that.

The funeral was lovely in every way, the reading that my sister and I did was heartfelt, genuine and true from the three of us children. The turnout was just perfect. He was a well liked and respected man and will be sorely missed.

The next three months were pretty good, I saw another side to Mother and I slowly let my guard down and allowed her into my heart. Sadly, it all changed again. I am sure as at some level she felt me open up and the old ways came back into her behaviour almost overnight. I became a replacement for Dad, her quiet anger directed at me. I was really hurting from being the subject of emotional attack and blackmail again and not in a good space at all to deal with it.

Moving on

I hadn't had time to reflect or grieve for Dad, as after the funeral, the focus was back onto mother and her needs. Work had become really busy and space for 'me time' was limited, in fact, almost non existent. I was tired, tetchy and craved peace and space. I couldn't make any sound decisions about the future or get back in touch with any dreams I may have for my life. I was closed down and worried about mother's future and how she would cope if I wasn't around. The fears were tangible. Time to do something about it, time to create some space and time to heal.

I planned a long trip away, a test for both of us really. I did my best to prepare Mum in practical terms by building support around her whilst I was to be away. My brother was going to keep an eye on her during this time away and my sister would phone regularly from Ireland and her best friend would drive her around if need be. The neighbours were a Godsend too.

It was a testing time, as I took a long flight to the island of Kaua'i for a five week trip. I would be on the other side of the world, away from everything and not so easy to get back quickly. I let go. I wanted no contact with the family and gave them instructions to call me only if it was absolutely necessary. I said my goodbyes to mother, both verbally and internally with forgiveness and love, knowing that if anything happened whilst I was a way, I had a clear heart and blessing from my brother and sister.

I felt like I had been in a desert during this particular period with my parents, marking time in my own world, feeling miles apart from what was theirs. I would never have been able to be there for my Mum and Dad had I not gained the strength necessary through my life experiences. I had come a long way from that frightened very shy little girl. The further I travelled away from the UK, the stronger the memories and feelings from previous trips to Hawaii came flooding back. I felt like I was being replenished and all the anxieties and deeply sad times were melting away.

I had a fabulous time in Hawaii. I was on retreat; a light, detox alkaline diet of delicious fresh vegetarian food, great meditations and the opportunity to visit some very special places including the island of Ni'ihau. We even experienced the alarm of a tsunami, this time with proper warning sirens and evacuation plans in place. Fortunately, the tsunami missed the island of Kaua'i, however the Big Island was not so lucky and suffered some structural damage, but no lives were lost.

Old patterns return

I came back from my trip, feeling strong and infinitely more aligned. The magic of the islands had yet again worked wonders for my soul, body and mind. When I returned, I realised I needn't have worried.

Mother proved to us all, including herself, that she could cope and had actually learned to enjoy space on her own.

Now with a renewed sense of self and direction, I started to look for somewhere to live. First though, I was very worried about our little dog Susie. She wasn't well and we took her to the vets. Mother wanted her put down, however, I knew deep down she wasn't ready. The vet couldn't find anything wrong with her and she was still eating and drinking. The vet put it down to a virus and slowly after a week, she got her sparkle back and looked forward to her morning walks with me again.

As Susie got better, mother got worse and slipped back into her old pattern of behaviour with me. It was like she had forgotten who she was again whilst I wasn't around and became demanding, dependant and unwilling to take any real responsibility. I found it extremely difficult to deal with and realised I had to get out sooner rather than later as the situation was killing me too.

By a series of synchronistic events I found an idyllic apartment not far from work and not too far from mother. I craved space, my own space and the apartment was perfect. It was surrounded by countryside, quiet, peaceful and large. All manner of countryside animals were in abundance and in full view, deer, foxes, sheep and rabbits to name but a few.

I was anxious about breaking the news to mother as although we had discussed me moving out before I went away, I knew she would become fearful and take it the wrong way. True to form, she became angry and hateful, yet she clearly didn't want me around either. I stood my ground, through the most challenging time and went ahead with arrangements to move out.

Guilt would flood through me every now and then as I wondered how mother would be living on her own, yet I had a deep knowing that I had to move out. My emotions became raw as I battled with the feelings and thoughts around the whole situation. One minute I was thinking this would be the best move for both of us and the next experiencing feelings of worry about mother. I was also conscious of the need to let go for good all the angst that had been created in my parent's home environment over the years as well as letting go of Dad's connection and his imprint that had been left on the home. I had to keep in mind that Mother had proved that she could live on her own, a fact that had been confirmed by my sister who, because she was away from the situation, could see clearly that me moving out was the best for both of us. Mother was not going to let me go without creating a full blown drama, I knew that. What I didn't know was what form that would take.

As the weeks went by, getting nearer to me moving out mother became communicative again and started looking forward to getting her home into order once I had left. She became almost impatient for me to go. On the weekend I was due to move out, I picked up the keys to my new home and decided to show mother as she had been pleasant to be with during the previous two weeks. I showed her round my new apartment and slowly saw her change. She became quiet and withdrawn and I realised she was jealous. I had seen that reaction before so I knew I was in for a rough ride. I knew I had to stay emotionally disengaged from her as much as I possibly could.

Come Monday morning it was time for me to go, and true to form mother could not bring herself to be civil. I went to give her a hug when I left but it was not well received. So I left with a heavy heart, trying my best to look forward, yet now anxious about mother, knowing she was in one of her rages.

Later that day, I had just put my dinner into the oven when the phone rang. It was mother in a state. The washing machine had flooded the kitchen. She wanted me to go back over and have a look.

"Could next door have a look for you," I said.

"No, I don't want to ask him."

"What about Dad's friend Ray over the road?"

"No he won't come."

All my suggestions went on deaf ears. I told her I had just put my dinner on and she promptly said, "I thought you would have." This made me even more suspicious, as she knew it wasn't a good time for me to drop everything and come over.

Too exhausted to battle anymore, I went over. Mother obviously wanted someone to fight with. It seemed she hated me, the dog and indeed, everyone. There I was taking the brunt of it all. I stayed as unemotional as I could and talked in practical terms about getting the machine fixed. I did what I needed to do to calm the situation down. After I had ordered a new part online and told her my brother would fix the new seal, I took my leave. She didn't even say thank you or goodbye when I left.

I went back to my new home annoyed with myself for just dropping everything again to run over to mother and spent some time beating myself up over the whole situation.

Slowly over the next few days I began to realise why I had had to move out. I would come home into my own space, thoroughly enjoying the solitude. It was so different to come home to clear energy with no anxiety about what mood I would find mother in. I found myself revelling in the bliss of it all.

The weekend arrived. I had been in my new home for exactly five days. It was time to take mother shopping, I dreaded meeting her, wondering what I would find. As I walked into the lounge, she was smiling and happy - what a transformation. She had had a lovely week. On one of the days my Aunt had taken her out, much of the rest of the time she had been in the garden, thoroughly enjoying herself. Nothing was said about the washing machine, it was as if it hadn't happened. My nephew and his new baby were coming to stay with her for the weekend. Phew! I took her shopping and waited for my nephew to arrive. I spent some time catching up with him, then took my leave and went home. What a relief, mother is going to be okay!

The next day I was due to go to work. I had just arrived when I realised I had some missed calls on my cell phone from my nephew. I called him back and was shocked to hear that mother had fallen over whilst they were taking the dog out for a walk and she was currently being seen into the ambulance! I couldn't believe the timing of it all!

My nephew couldn't stay as he had a long drive back home with the baby. So, off I went again. I left work and went straight to the scene and followed mother to A & E. She had dislocated her shoulder, and broken a bone in her foot. My Sunday was spent at the hospital with her. I ended up staying overnight. It was a miserable thing to have happened to her at this stage. I must say mother was very brave and stayed cheerful throughout the time.

Mother had said that Susie had been off her food. My heart sank as mother told me that she had made the decision to have her put down. I was heartbroken. She was the last link to my Dad and the only one, apart from Dad, who received my love. Mother had been complaining about Susie for months. She didn't want to take care of the dog and had no real connection with her. Neither myself nor my brother were in a position to have her. She was an old dog of fifteen years, even though she still looked like a puppy and was the sweetest little animal you could ever wish for.

Our little dog was always admired by everyone when we took her out on a walk. There was not a nasty bone in her body and she was full of character. Exactly a week later, following mother's adamant instructions, my brother and I took her to the vets. The night before I sobbed my heart out. I didn't sleep and thought I would never stop crying. The vet was running late, so we decided to see if she wanted a little walk. All of a sudden she came alive, revelling in smelling the grass. I started to doubt if this was right. As I picked her up again I could tell she was breathing heavily and the walk had been a struggle. She was very happy for me to carry her, confirming that this was actually the right thing to do.

The vet was brilliant. I hugged Susie in my arms. She sensed I was upset and stuck to me like a magnet. I felt awful. I held her little face in my hands and looked directly into her eyes as the injection was delivered to put her to sleep. It was heartbreaking. I scattered her ashes in the same place as Dads knowing he would have liked that.

With Susie gone and me having moved out, mother now has no reminders of Dad apart from her own memories of him. She seems happy for now, her bones are healing and she appears to relish her own space. My hope is that she will find some true peace and happiness and find herself in a more manageable place. My brother and I continue to support the best we can. My relationship with her is functional, as I choose not to open myself up knowing that she thinks and feels differently to the rest of the family. This is the legacy of mental illness, distorted even more so by a lifetime of prescription drugs. When you are born into it and have had to live with it, it's even more difficult to see your way clearly and create healthy boundaries.

Full circle

What an adventure. I feel like I have literally done a full circle. Nothing has changed, except within myself, where everything has changed. Now, yet again, I have become consciously aware of what is being played out with my mother and can choose whether or not to engage.

I am grateful that I have learned to live and love without fear and follow my heart's desire. I could have easily shut down, ending up trapped in fear over the years. However, I tried that and was woken up again, many times. I don't regret a thing. Strength comes from within, if you let it shine through. I continue to spend time in my spiritual home of Hawaii when I can and currently live in the UK. My dreams come alive every day, as I trust in 'the all that is.' I have learned to let go, forgive and more importantly trust in myself with guidance from the Divine.

Other titles from MasterWorks International

Available from
www.masterworksinternational.com
and all good bookstores

Quinta-Essentia
by Morag Campbell
A study of the Five Natural Elements and.how they all affect our lives even today.

A Promise Kept
by Morag Campbell
Autobiographical account of a profound spiritual adventure set in England and ancient Hawaii.

The Power of Love - A Guide to Consciousness and Change
by Phil Young and Morag Campbell
The ancient Polynesian viewpoint on spiritual development retold for the modern world.

The Way of the FlameKeeeper
by David Kala Ka La
A no punches pulled account of a personal spiritual journey

Polarity Therapy - Healing with Life Energy
by Alan Siegel ND and Phil Young
A clear extensively illustrated instruction manual in this unique healing art of energy balancing..

Earthkind
by Morag Campbell
There is something for everyone in this light-hearted fairy tale with a strong ecological theme

The Art of Mental Wellbeing - The Polarity Of Mental Wellbeing and Mental Disorder beyond the Medical Approach
by Tony Caves
An exploration of sacred geometry and energy in relation to mental health.

Mindessence - The Polarity of Life and Death
by Tony Caves
Ideas and methods to move beyond the notion of Life and Death and realise our true nature.

Sink the Relation Ship - Transform the Way you Relate
by Morag Campbell
A humorous, yet hard hitting look, at the problems that arise as a result of the way that we think about relationships. Contains practical suggestions for improving the way we relate.

Resistance - The Whole Truth
by Celia Jennings
Resistance is humourously explored as it apertains to Science, Metaphysics, Biology and Spirituality

Dont'Start What You Can't Finish
by Morag Campbell
Another humorous, yet hard hitting look, at the importance of completing things in life with strategies you can adopt to get the job done.